CONTRIBUTORS:

1. Associate Professor Ivan Manchev, MD, PhD

Head of the department of Neurology and Psyhiatry at the faculty of Medicine, Thracian University, Stara Zagora, Bulgaria

2. Professor Ivan Georgiev, Medical University, Sofia, Bulgaria

Systemic Hereditary Degenerative and Dystrophic Diseases of the Nervous and Muscular System

by

Ivan Manchev

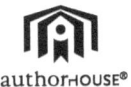
authorHOUSE®

AuthorHouse™ UK Ltd.
500 Avebury Boulevard
Central Milton Keynes, MK9 2BE
www.authorhouse.co.uk
Phone: 08001974150

First published by AuthorHouse 11/26/2007

ISBN: 978-1-4343-4644-5 (sc)

Library of Congress Control Number: 2007908445

Printed in the United States of America
Bloomington, Indiana

This book is printed on acid-free paper.

SYSTEMIC HEREDITARY DEGENERATIVE AND DYSTROPHIC DISEASES OF THE NERVOUS AND MUSCULAR SYSTEM

Ass. prof. Ivan Manchev, M.D.

Hereditary degenerative and dystrophic disorders of the nervous system and the neuromuscular apparatus represent a field of medicine which conjugates the interests of neurologists, psychiatrists, pediatricians and other specialists, as well as general physicians. The interest for these diseases has increased, especially during the past few years due to the progress of the fundamental genetic investigations. Population genetics has demonstrated the prevalence of many of these disorders, as well as the pattern of their monogenic inheritance. A number of biochemical markers – participants in the pathogenesis of these diseases - have been found, which are used for diagnostics. A number of new hereditary syndromes and disorders have been differentiated. Large studies including DNA-analysis with mapping of pathologic genes, carriers of these diseases, are currently being conducted. These data reveal broad perspectives for early diagnosis, carrier identification and prophylaxis. They also outline some possibilities for therapeutic effects.

There are a few publications on hereditary neurological diseases in literature. The proposed handbook is directed mainly towards diagnostics, differential diagnosis, contemporary measures for treatment and prophylaxis.

INTRODUCTION

Dramatic progress has been achieved in the field of medical genetics, molecular biology and electron microscopy during the last few decades. This has led to an improvement of the diagnostic, prophylactic and therapeutic measures for genetic disorders and malformations as for the screening, covering the heterozygotes, prenatal diagnostics, gene mapping, DNA-analysis of mutations, etc. Certain progress has also been reached in the treatment and quality of life of these patients. Yet the results of the therapeutic achievements remain unsatisfactory. There is no uniform agreement about classification and precise clinical connotation of the separate nosological units. In the present work an attempt for such a summary will be made. /35/

According to etiology there are 4 groups of hereditary disorders:

- monogenic disorders: over 3 300 different mutations are known, which are divided into autosomal dominant /1 800/, autosomal recessive /1 300/, and X-linked /240/ according to the type of inheritance;
- polygenic disorders: they are the result of the effect of numerous genes and environmental factors, which are unidentified in most cases;
- chromosomal abnormalities: associated with alterations in the usual number or structure of the chromosomes;
- teratogenic abnormalities: they occur as a result of exogenous and endogenous factors acting during embryogenesis;

CHARACTERISTICS OF THE MONOGENIC AND POLYGENIC TYPE OF INHERITANCE

1. Monogenic type of inheritance.

The three classical types of inheritance /75/ are presented on fig. 1.

1.1 Autosomal dominant type of inheritance.

Mutation of one of the allelic genes /heterozygosity/ is sufficient to cause the phenotype / due to the low incidence of dominant mutations, homozygosity is practically not observed/. Variable expressivity refers to variable phenotypic manifestation, e.g. more or less expressed, early or late onset of the disease, frequently among one family members also. The term reduced penetrance is used to describe the absence of any clinical signs in a relative despite the fact that he is also a heterozygote. In other cases the first occurrence of a disease with established dominant pattern of inheritance indicates a new mutation or a nongenetic phenocopy.

1.2 Autosomal recessive type of inheritance.

Relatives are affected only in case two copies of the mutant gene are present /homozygosity/. This happens only if both parents are heterozygotes. The rarer the gene is among the population, the greatest the chance is that the parents are consanguineous.

1.3 X-linked inheritance.

It is usually recessive and sometimes dominant. Only males are affected by X-linked recessive disorders. when the disorder is genetically lethal /that is the patients do not reach reproductive age/, the inheritance occurs via the heterozygote mothers /carriers/ on half of their sons /e.g. Duchenne muscular dystrophy/. In cases of nonlethal and semilethal disorders all sons in the offspring of male patients are healthy, whereas all daughters are carriers. In sporadic cases sometimes there are new mutations and sometimes the mothers are also carriers. Testing for heterozygosity is very important in X-linked inheritance. In the somatic cells of the carriers only one X-chromosome is genetically active, which can be either the one with the mutation or the normal one. The reason for this is in the inactivation of one of the X-chromosomes during the early embryonic phase /Lyan's hypothesis/. As this process begins very early and is random, the relative portion of cells in the adult with normal and mutant X-chromosome, respectively, is extremely variable. This is the reason why it is never possible to include all carriers in heterozygote testing.

2. Polygenic type of inheritance.

The development of a significant number of malformations is clearly the result of the effects of several genes and different other hereditary factors /multifactorial etiology/. The associated risks for inheritance in the patient's relatives differ significantly from the monogenic type of inheritance. The reason for this includes the following factors:

-   the incidence of the anomaly among population;
-   the degree of manifestation of the disorder in the investigated individual;
-   the degree of relation between the investigated individual and the person at risk;
-   the gender of the investigated individual and the person at risk;
-   the number of cases already established in the family;
-   the observed differences in the concordance in identical and nonidentical twins.

On the basis of this the risk in each family should be assessed individually.

Hereditary degenerative disorders are transmitted genetically and affect one or several parts of the central nervous system. Because of this they are classified according to the anatomic localization of the defects.

INHERITANCE /PEDIGREE PATTERN/CHARACTERISTICS

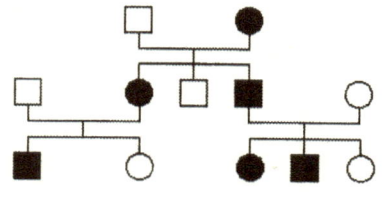

- it is inherited by 50% of the
  children of an affected parent;
- males and females are equally
  affected;
- variable expressivity in most
  cases;

Autosomal dominant

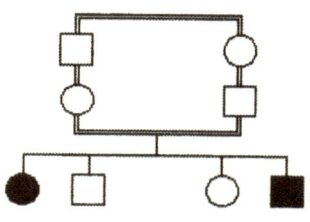

- it is inherited by 25% of the
  children of two healthy
  heterozygous parents;
- males and females are equally
  affected;
- consanguinity is frequently
  encountered;

Autosomal recessive

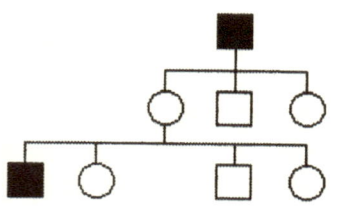

- only male individuals are affected;
  - patients' offspring:
    all sons are healthy,
    all daughters are healthy
    heterozygous carriers;
  - carriers' offspring:
    50% of the sons are affected,
    50% of the daughters are carriers;

X-linked

Fig. 1 The three classic types of inheritance.

Chapter I

DYSTROPHIC DISORDERS OF THE BRAIN WITH PREDOMINANT LOCALIZATION IN THE CORTEX AND DEMENTIA SYNDROMES

The contemporary development of neuroscience has led to significant improvement in diagnostic and therapeutic methods in the field of the most topical neurological conditions: the cerebrovascular disorders. The problem of dementia in late and presenile age has drawn great interest during the last decades.

The issue, concerning presenile dementia affecting people in active age and leading to early loss of work capacity and to intellectual and work deficit, is of great importance. This makes the problem with their expedient diagnostics social, as well as medical. Presenile dementias are endogenous, primary dystrophic and progressive conditions in which focal neurological symptoms and syndromes of variable severity are observed along with dementia manifestations.

1. Alzheimer's Disease
It is a primary degenerative neurological disorder of unknown origin. There exist a presenile form /type II/ and a senile form /type I/. In the contemporary classification of dementia /International Classification of Diseases – 10, ch. V/ the former "senile and presenile dementias" is now substituted for Alzheimer's Disease /4/.

Frequency. This disorder represents a dramatic medico-social problem. It begins after 40 years of age and rarely earlier. It

1

usually occurs between 55 and 65 years of age. 5 to 10 % of cases occur in this age group and approximately 20 %: over the age of 80. Females are more susceptible than males and the total duration of the illness is from 2 to 10 years. Alzheimer's Disease is assumed to be the cause of approximately 50 % of dementias.

Etiology and pathogenesis. Unknown. The disease usually occurs sporadically but a genetic relation is also supposed. In familial forms /approximately 10-15%/ it presents as a monogenic disorder inherited in autosomal dominant pattern. The locus of the pathologic gene was found in chromosome 21 /patients with Down syndrome – trisomy 21 – develop similar changes in the brain and dementia/. There is data indicating genetic polymorphism: a DNA-marker has been found in chromosome 19 as well in a subgroup of patients with late onset of disease, as well as another gene locus in chromosome 14 in cases with early onset. A slow viral infection has been discussed for sometime now. The role of Aluminum intoxication in cases of Zinc deficiency has also been considered. Disturbed Aluminum metabolism is also found in dialysis dementia. Disturbances in the metabolism of all neurotransmitter systems and mostly of the cholinergic and noradrenergic system play an undoubtful role in the pathogenesis. In the brain of patients with Alzheimer's Disease the level of somatostatin, vasopressin, endorphins, substance P, etc. is also changed.

Pathomorphology. Generalized brain atrophy is found with a 15% reduction of the brain mass, mainly the cortex and particularly the frontal and parietal lobes. There is reduction of the neuronal population mainly in the hippocampus, substantia innominata and locus coeruleus. Intracellularly deposited spiral-like fibres /"neurofibrillar plexuses, corpuscles"/ are seen as well as extracellular deposition of lipoid, surrounded by dystrophically altered neurons /"neuronal plaques, senile plaques"/. It has recently been found that amyloid is deposited in the walls of brain vessels and A4 amyloid protein plays a role in plaque formation. The gene encoding the formation of these proteins is also localized in chromosome 21. A neurochemical sign, characteristic of the disease, is the marked decrease in the level of the enzyme acetylcholine esterase.

Clinical manifestations. Initial symptoms depend on the localization in the frontal or parietal lobes of the cortex. Symptoms usually develop gradually and silently. Critical thinking begins to fade first; the patient is attributing this to age. Often patients do not have obvious complaints, but are upset by the fact that they cannot answer simple questions, and then history is gathered from family members. Spontaneousness and initiativeness are lost early in the disease course. The patient gives up his/her usual activities and loses the relationship with the social surroundings. There are disturbances in the fixation memory; the patients cannot remember new names; they have difficulty finding the appropriate words. At these stage memory impairment is more often related to recent events. The patient can maintain an elementary conversation with his/her relatives and friends but he/she loses this ability in unfamiliar surroundings. Patients' interests gradually narrow to a phase of affective stupor. Depressive states may occur which sometimes alter with agitation and anxiety. Examination of patients in the initial stage of the disease usually reveals disturbance of the memory for recent events and a variable degree of cognitive deficit. Oral automatisms may be seen. In the late stages of the disease unexplainable omissions in everyday activities /at work and at home/ are observed; the patient's looks and personal hygiene are being neglected. Space disorientation increases especially in unfamiliar environment. Apathy or unprovoked irritability and aggression are observed. Memory impairment, speech and behavioral disturbances increase to an extent that the patients can no longer take care of themselves. They are anxious, nervous and often lose their way when left alone, especially at night. Their speech becomes nonspontaneous and uneven, aphasic mistakes are encountered, there are difficulties in understanding more complex instructions. Transcortical motor aphasia is more pronounced in young patients. Kinetic and constructive apraxia and agnosia may be observed.

In the late stages of mental symptoms increase, psychoses and paranoia occur, as well as stupor, delirium and insanity with more severe forms. Disorientation in all spheres becomes more pronounced; logic thinking, combination skills and semantic relations are severely impaired. Frequently epileptic seizures develop.

Neurological examination does not find spastic pareses, pathologic hyperreflexia, pathologic reflexes or oral automatisms. Parkinson's syndrome with rigidity, bradykinesia and tremor is observed frequently. Severe apraxia, mutism and incontinence develop in terminal stages of the disease. Patients become entirely handicapped by severe contractures. Cases with disease onset before 65 years of age, which are more often familial, progress faster and more symptoms originating from the frontal and parietal lobe /aphasias and apraxias/ are found at objective neurological examination.

Diagnosis and differential diagnosis. Diagnosis is usually not difficult to make in cases of manifested symptoms of the disease in young people and lack of risk factors for development of other types of dementia. Psychological testing for diagnosis of "global" dementias is obligatory. Computer tomography /CT/ and Magnetic resonance imaging /MRI/ of the brain demonstrate cortical atrophy, explicitly pronounced in the frontal and parietal lobe and ventricular dilatation. Similar changes are found, however, with many other disorders, thus these alterations cannot be considered characteristic of the disease. Unfortunately in most cases Alzheimer's Disease has to be distinguished mainly from other types of dementia with similar course. Since the diagnosis can be certain only with histological examination of a biopsy specimen and this is practically very hard to perform, one should be well aware the clinical manifestations of the following diseases:

A. In the early stage of the disease.

A.1. Depressive Syndrome. Pseudodementia in Depression.
Depression is a condition which is often mistaken for dementia. Thus there differentiation is of clinical importance. Dementia and pseudodementia in depression share some common features: slowed thinking, apathy, irritability, memory and concentration impairment, behavioral and personality changes. Besides in some cases dementia may coexist with depression. There are, however, a number of differences between the two conditions: the onset of dementia is gradual, with progressive worsening, whereas the onset of depression is abrupt. In dementia there is no past history of depressive changes, whereas in depression

there is such a history. In dementia patients are not aware of the mental alterations and do not complain of memory impairment, whereas patients with depression are aware of these changes and tend to exaggerate their complaints of memory disturbance. In dementia there no somatic complaints, whereas there are such in depression; in the first case autonomic symptoms are weak and in the second case: they are manifest. Neurologic examination and laboratory tests in dementia usually demonstrate pathologic changes, whereas there are no such in depression.

A.2. The Symptom of Amnesia.

Amnesia is a time-limited or content-limited memory deficit that can occur because of organic changes or functional disturbances. Damage to the brain structures leads to time-limited memory blanks. To the contrary, emotional stress and unpleasant events can be a reason for content-limited memory blanks. They can develop in healthy individuals also.

Organically induced and time-limited syndromes of amnesia can occur as either acute or chronic. Acute amnesias are observed with acute alterations in the state of consciousness, cranial trauma, cerebral ischemia /mostly in cases of bilateral infarction in the area supplied by the posterior cerebral artery/, alcohol intoxication, Wernicke's encephalopathy, etc. syndromes of amnesia can also develop chronically: in Korsakoff's alcohol amnestic syndrome, following encephalitis, in cases of brain tumors, as a paraneoplastic syndrome, etc.

There are several types of amnestic syndromes:

    a) transient global amnesia; Most frequent in elderly people. It presents with transient and complete inability to remember. It is characterized by suddenly occurring limited ability or complete inability to remember past days or weeks with preserved time and space orientation. It usually follows a reverse course but there are also cases of permanent amnestic blanks.

b) retrograde amnesia; Patients with retrograde amnesia are unable to recall the last events preceding the trauma. The duration of the retrograde amnesia can be used for estimating the severity of the trauma. The duration of amnesia, however, is not proportional to the severity and duration of the period of altered consciousness. Retrograde amnesia may be short-lived regardless a long period of unconsciousness.

c) anterograde amnesia; This term is used to indicate loss of memory for events following the trauma and regain of consciousness which is due to inability to fixate and preserve memory traits.

d) Korsakoff's amnestic syndrome; This is a typical amnestic syndrome. It develops most often in cases of chronic ethylism, following Wernicke's encephalopathy, carbon dioxide poisoning and severe cranial trauma. Amnesia, disorientation, confabulations, impaired ability for comprehension, euphoria, lack of critical reasoning and sometimes passivity are very of the clinical course of the syndrome. The neurologic examination reveals ophthalmoplegia, impaired coordination, extrapyramidal symptoms, various dyskinesias, tone alterations, epileptic seizures and alterations in consciousness, as well as frequent polyneuritic syndrome.

B. During the late stage of the disease one should consider:

B.1. Vascular Dementia

The term multiinfarction dementia refers to dementia associated with large cerebral infarctions. It most frequently includes fluctuant psychopathological changes. The term vascular dementia is more appropriate in order to cover the whole spectrum of dementias occurring in cerebrovascular disease /CVD/. Vascular dementia is defined as reduction in the cognitive abilities of a patient with CVD when compared to the initial level. Characteristic clinical manifestations of vascular dementia usually develop after 50 years of age. This dementia is due to multiple small and usually neurologically "silent" foci of liquification in both cerebral hemispheres. Its pathomorphologic substrate is loss of neurons and axons. The severity of the clinical manifestations is dependent on the total area of these small infarctions.

The onset of the disease is usually abrupt, with a fluctuant course. Memory is preserved for a relatively long period; in the beginning there are no personality changes yet. Emotional disturbances with affective lability and uncontrollability, as well as paranoic ideas and delirium experiences are frequently encountered. Abstract thinking is narrowed and judgment is impaired. Focal neurologic signs develop gradually: dysarthria, dysphagia, small-step gait, aphasias, apraxias, pyramidal and extrapyramidal symptoms.

To establish the diagnosis of vascular dementia the presence of memory disturbances together with several cognitive disturbances /attention, speech, orientation, critical reasoning, praxis, motor control/, found at clinical examination and objectivized via psychological testing, is required. Finding cerebrovascular stenoses and thromboses via Doppler sonography, brain infarctions and atrophy via computer tomography and MRI is of great significance. Single photon emission computed tomography and even cerebral angiography is performed if required. Reological properties of the blood and the condition of the cardiovascular system are tested.

2. Creutzfeldt-Jacob Disease.

Synonyms. Jacob's spastic pseudosclerosis, abiotrophic dementia, cortico-strio-spinal degeneration.

A typical example of slow viral transmissive encephalopathies with an invariably fatal outcome which is characterized by progressive dementia and variable symptoms originating from the cortex, basal ganglia, cerebellum and spinal cord. The disease is encountered in all continents and sometimes exhibits a genetic trait. Its frequency is 1: 1,000,000 of the population. It is found in patients from 20 to 80 years of age, but most frequently between 50 and 74 years of age; both genders are equally affected. Spongious dystrophy with astroglial proliferation as foci, localized in the cerebral cortex, the cerebellum, the basal ganglia, the medulla oblongata and the spinal cord are found pathomorphologically. Senile plaques and vascular changes are absent in contrast to Alzheimer's Disease.

One of the cardinal symptoms of the disease is presenile dementia which includes memory impairment, disorientation, confusion and intellectual deficit. Mental changes, such as anxiety, euphoria, depression, hallucinations, personality degradation, are apparent. Objective neurologic examination reveals pyramidal and extrapyramidal symptoms such as pareses, spastic rigidity, tremor, dysarthria, athetosis, etc. Manifestations of Parkinsonism may also be observed. In terminal stages severe impairment of consciousness such as akinetic mutism and coma are noted. Electroencephalographic investigation /EEG/ shows stereotypically repetitive paroxysms of sharp waves or spikes with a background activity of slow delta- and theta-waves.

Patients come to a lethal end within 1.5 to 2 years.

3. AIDS Dementia Complex.

AIDS-dementia is progressive dementia associated with motor functional and behavioral problems. AIDS encephalopathy, AIDS subacute encephalitis or AIDS related dementia are related to this term. These complications from the nervous system are found in approximately 70% of patients. AIDS dementia complex is a result from direct invasion of the HIV retrovirus into the brain tissue. Severe cortical atrophy with massive neuronal death, microglial expansion, astrogliosis and marked perivenous demielinization are found pathomorphologically in the patients' brains. White matter, basal ganglia, thalamus, pons and spinal cord are gradually involved.

Clinically AIDS dementia complex is manifested with general malaise, progressive memory fading, depressive states, apathic behavior, sometimes hallucinations. Patients suffer attention deficit, they become confused and disoriented. The objective neurologic examination finds cerebellar ataxia, pyramidal signs such as pathologic hyperreflexia and the presence of pathologic reflexes, tremor and dysarthria. Muscle rigidity, urinary and/or fecal incontinence, myoclonic movements, oral automatisms, epileptic seizures, tetraplegia and deterioration of the mental symptoms, sometimes visual hallucinations are observed in advanced stages of the disease.

The diagnosis is established via virus investigation. Different from Alzheimer's Disease, mononuclear pleocytosis, increased level of the CSF protein over 200 mg/dl, decreased level of glucose and oligiclonal curve type with increased immunoglobulin G at electrophoresis are found in the CSF of patients with AIDS dementia complex. Computer tomography and magnetic resonance imaging demonstrate cortical atrophy and lesions in the white matter of the brain. Patients die of Pneumocystic pneumonia or peritonitis following bowel perforation approximately one or two years after the full manifestation of the disease.

4. Progressive Paralysis.

Progressive paralysis is a chronic inflammatory disease in the late stage of inadequately treated syphilis. The disorder presents mainly with mental symptoms and develops approximately 10 – 20 years after the infection. Approximately 5 – 10% of patients with syphilis develop the manifestations of progressive paralysis with predominance of males. Panencephalitis with subsequent brain atrophy is found pathomorphologically. Basal ganglia are subsequently involved. Clinical manifestations include mental and neurologic symptoms. The most characteristic signs of the mental ones is expansive mania-like syndrome which presents as megalomania with overestimation of oneself and nonsensical and exaggerated ideas of grandeur. Progressive paralysis begins with a pseudoneurasthenic syndrome, loss of fixation memory, attention deficit and sleep disturbances. Severe dementia develops, sometimes combined with euphoria. Objective neurologic examination reveals positive Argyll-Robertson symptom, areflexia, impaired deep sensitivity, ataxia, positive Romberg sign, incontinence, impotence, deformity of the knees "genu recurvatum" type, etc.

The diagnosis is established with the aid of specific serological tests for confirming syphilis. The prognosis is unfavorable.

5. Parkinson's Disease.

Patients with Parkinsonism often develop manifestations of dementia, especially in more advanced stages of the disease. This is especially true for cases in which Parkinson's Syndrome develops following a vascular or postencephalic damage. On the other hand Alzheimer's Disease can also be complicated with signs of Parkinsonism. In both cases, however, the differential diagnosis is based on the symptom complex characteristic of Parkinson's Disease which is never so demonstrative in Alzheimer's Disease, on the history data for another major previous disease and the beneficial clinical response to antiparkinson drugs, which is not seen in Alzheimer's Disease. Psychological tests, which support the diagnosis of Alzheimer's Disease, are also of great importance. Furthermore even in the beginning of Alzheimer's Disease mental symptoms are prevalent, whereas in Parkinsonism these symptoms usually progress slowly for a period of several years.

6. Pick's Disease.

In contrast to Alzheimer's Disease, Pick's Disease begins at an earlier age /around the 4th decade/. Personality disturbances are leading among mental problems and cognitive disturbances, characteristic of Alzheimer's Disease, appear not before the terminal stages of the disorder. In Pick's Disease focal neurologic symptoms are much more discreet and when they develop, they are characterized by frontal lobe syndrome.

7. Huntington's Chorea.

It begins at an earlier age /most often between 25 and 45 years of age/ in comparison with Alzheimer's Disease. Alterations in the affective sphere, attention and sensory disturbances, memory fading, hypochondric and hypodepressive syndromes predominate among the mental disturbances. The appearance of choreic hyperkinesias as large, rapid, involuntary movements, occurring tumultuously in different muscle groups is typical. In such instances differentiation of Huntington's Chorea from Alzheimer's Disease does not present a difficulty.

8. Hepatocerebral Dystrophy.

The coexistence of dementia with extrapyramidal disturbances predominates in its clinical course. To the contrary of Alzheimer's Disease, Hepatocerebral Dystrophy develops mainly in young people. Most often the first symptom is tremor which affects mainly the upper extremities. Various extrapyramidal hyperkinesias develop such as chorea, athetosis, torion dystonia, etc. Hepatic lesions and the typical green corneal ring of Kaiser-Fleischer are characteristic of the disease, which are not present in Alzheimer's Disease. Low serum level of copper and increased excretion of copper with urine are also noted. In this case dementia goes together with mental retardation, attention deficit and severe memory impairment.

Evolution. In the initial stages of the disease patients cope with their professional and everyday duties relatively well. The disease, however, gradually progresses and these patients become a serious medical and social issue. In advanced countries they need constant medical attention. Death occurs in 5 to 10 years since the appearance of the first symptoms.

Treatment. For now there is no drug effective enough to stop disease progression. Several drugs with vasodilatator effect /Papaverine, Dihydroergotoxine/ are used, as well as central nervous system stimulants /amphetamines, Pentilentetrazol, Procainamide/, neuropeptides /Vasopresin/, opium antagonists / Naloxone/, but their effect is unsatisfactory. Due to the impairment of cholinergic neuronal systems and depletion of acetylcholine transferase in the brain of patients with Alzheimer's Disease, attempts are conducted for affecting the disorder in this direction. Acetylcholine precursors /choline, lecitin/, drugs stimulating the release of acetylcholine /Piracetam, 4-aminopyridine, Tacrine/ and agonists of the muscarinic cholinergic receptors /arecholine/ are administered experimentally.

Prophylaxis. It is not very effective at present. Early diagnosis and treatment can to some extent slow disease progression but results are unsatisfactory.

9. Pick's Disease.

A degenerative disease characterized by slow progression and development of dementia and neurologic symptoms mainly from the frontal lobe.

Its incidence is 4-5 times lower than that of Alzheimer's Disease. It affects women approximately twice more often than men. It has high genetic predisposition and most often develops after the 4th decade.

Etiology and pathogenesis. Not known.

Pathomorphology. Most frequently it affects the frontal lobe followed by the temporal lobe. Neuronal death and glial expansion is found in the cortex. Here there are no senile plaques or Alzheimer neurofibrils in contrast to Alzheimer's Disease.

Clinical manifestations. Similar to Alzheimer's Disease, Pick's Disease has a slow and imperceptible course, progressing without fluctuations. Mental changes predominate: personality changes with loss of the sense of tact with increasing sense of distance, whereas cognitive functions are preserved for a relatively long period of time. Loss of inhibitions and criminal behavior are noticed. There is affective lability and sleep disturbance. Memorization and orientation are gradually affected. Loss of moral values and ignorance of professional and family duties are frequently observed.

Neurologic symptomatics is relatively less pronounced. Frontal ataxia, motor aphasia, apraxia, Jacksonian motor seizures, etc., characteristic of frontal lobe disorder appear. Extrapyramidal manifestations with Parkinson's syndrome can also be observed. Attacks of cataplexy can also occur /25/.

Diagnosis and differential diagnosis. Diagnosis is made on the basis of the characteristic clinical course and confirmation of the dementia via psychological testing. Differential diagnosis is made with the same diseases as for Alzheimer's Disease. Treatment is also the same.

Prognosis. Unfavorable. Usually the disease progresses very quickly and leads to death in 2-3 years.

Prophylaxis. There are no effective prophylactic measures for now.

Chapter II

HEREDITARY DEGENERATIVE DISORDERS OF BASAL GANGLIA WITH PREDOMINANT EXTRAPYRAMIDAL SYNDROMES

1. Huntington's Chorea

A chronic progressive hereditary degenerative disorder characterized by increasing choreic hyperkinesias and dementia.

Synonyms. Hereditary chorea, chronic progressive chorea, choreic dementia.

Frequency. It is observed in all countries and populations with various frequency: from 30 to 70/ 1 000 000 people. It usually begins in middle age: between 25 and 45 years of age affecting males slightly more often than females.

Etiology and pathogenesis. The disorder is hereditary and is transmitted in autosomal dominant pattern, but cases with negative family history are not infrequent. Transmission occurs from affected parents. The pathologic gene associated with this disorder expresses high penetrance /80-85%/. Application of DNA-recombination method has made it possible to localize the pathologic gene in chromosome 4, which is of great importance in medicogenetic counseling and sets up prerequisites for working out an adequate therapeutic approach. Disturbances in brain metabolism and especially in the metabolism of different neurotransmitters and neuromodulators are considered to play an important role in the pathogenesis of the disease. The main symptoms of the disease develop due to marked degeneration of extrapyramidal GABAergic systems, increased functional activity of dopaminergic systems and decreased cholinergic activity. Insufficient level of GABA is found in cerebral neurons; the level of iron is increased in substantia nigra cells; and erythrocytes contain more manganese. Changes in the concentrations of neuropeptides in basal ganglia have been found: including decreased substance P, methionine, enkephalins, cholecystokinins, and the levels of somatostatin and neuropeptide Y are increased. Errors in oxidative metabolism are generally considered to be the basis of the disease /88/.

The mechanism of motor disorders has been studied. The reason for the lack of control over synergic movements and muscle tone by substantia nigra is the blockage of strionigral pathways. As a result substantia nigra passes on the information received from the premotor cortex to anterior root cells in a pulsative manner.

Brain atrophy is found pathomorphologically. Most affected are anterior cerebral lobes, striatum, substantia nigra, globus pallidus, in which neuronal death is seen. In the cerebellar cortex mainly Purkinje cells are damaged. Grossly the brain is reduced in size, the ventricles are dilated.

Clinical manifestations. There are several clinical familial variants: classic, Wesphal akinetic-rigid variant, juvenile variant, hereditary nonprogressive chorea and atypical variants.

In its classic variant the disease begins between 25 and 45 years of age. Hyperkinesias present as large, rapid, arrhythmic and involuntary movements, occurring tumultuously in different muscle groups. The patients grimace, gesticulate, the gait is broad-based, the arms are wide extended. As a result of that walking and writing become difficult. Hyperkinesias of speech muscles presents with slow, uneven speech which is accompanied by redundant sounds. Hyperkinesias increase with agitation and disappear during sleep. They can be of many different types: choreic, athetosic, dystonic, and sometimes they affect half of the body: hemichorea. Mental changes, which are the other major manifestation of the disorder, are presented as changes in the emotional sphere and with abrupt intellectual decline. Patients are emotionally unstable, irritable, and sometimes apathic. Hypochondric and hypodepressive syndromes are observed. Sometimes patients exhibit asocial behavior; suicidal attempts are not infrequent either. Intellect gradually declines, memory weakens, attention becomes difficult to concentrate, mental capacity is lost. Severe dementia develops with complete indifference to the surroundings and loss of all mental capacity.

Wesphal variant /akinetic-rigid variant/ is characterized by more slightly pronounced hyperkinesias at the expense of severe rigidity of the muscles of the lower legs and trunk; and in the terminal stages contractures develop.

The juvenile variant is found in approximately 50% of cases and begins in children younger than 15 years of age /anticipation phenomenon in children with affected parents/. The main symptoms in children are: hypokinesia, rigidity, epileptic seizures, mental degradation. Classic hyperkinesia or choreoathetosis is observed only in 30-50% of the patients and affects the head and proximal muscle groups. Cerebellar symptoms are seen more rarely.

Diagnosis and differential diagnosis. Positive family history is crucial for the diagnosis along with characteristic clinical manifestations. The differential diagnosis of classic chorea is made with senile chorea in patients with atherosclerosis. The major distinguishing feature in such cases is the absence of such condition in parents or other family members. Furthermore in these cases choreic hyperkinesias are more slightly pronounced and other symptoms are observed. Choreic syndrome can also develop in other diseases: tumors, encephalites, vascular disorders, etc. /14/. In these cases the course is different, there is no positive family history, symptoms related to the main disease are found, sometimes changes in CSF are noted. Chorea minor should be excluded in young people; it begins in childhood and is characterized by rapid increase in choreic hyperkinesias. This variant of chorea develops on the background of rheumatism and has a favorable course. In some cases one should consider hereditary cerebellar ataxia which is transmitted in an autosomal dominant pattern, as well as Alzheimer's Disease and Creutzfeldt-Jacob Disease. Extrapyramidal forceful movements can be observed with the latter two ones. They differ from Huntington's Chorea in the rapid progression of mental disturbances. Akinetic-rigid variant of Huntington's Chorea should be distinguished from hepatocerebral degeneration and torsion dystonia. Biochemical tests /impaired metabolism of Copper in hepatocerebral dystrophy/, as well as family history, are crucial in such cases. A loading dose of L-

DOPA can be used as a diagnostic test for the akinetic-rigid variant of the disease: choreic hyperkinesias appear or increase abruptly after taking the drug. The variants of the disease which go with marked mental symptoms in the absence of hyperkinesias should be differentiated from schizophrenia and other mental disorders. Finally, some conditions with symptomatic hyperkinesias: acute encephalitis, lupus erythematosus, leukodystrophies, hyperthyroidism, etc. have to be considered. Even more rarely, when seizures and mental retardation prevail, ceroidlipofuscinosis needs to be ruled out.

Evolution. The disease follows a slowly progressive course with intensification of rigidity, akinesia and mental disturbances in the final stages. The ability for active movement and caring for oneself is gradually lost. Severe cachexia develops.

Treatment. There is no etiologic therapy. Efforts are pointed at influencing choreic hyperkinesias. Antidopaminergic agents exhibit beneficial eefect. Neuroleptics are used: Haloperidol 3-6 mg/day; phenothiazines: Aminazine 150 mg/day, which blocks dopamine receptors. Apomorphine, which is an agonist of dopamine receptors, is used. Its favorable effect is explained with stimulation of presynaptic dopamine receptors which reduces the release of the mediator. Benzodiazepines have a beneficial effect on hyperkinesias. Stereoataxic surgery of basal ganglia can be applied in atypical variants /hemichorea, local choreoathetosis/. Small doses of L-DOPA /Madopar/ are noted to exert a positive effect in cases of akinetic-rigid variant.

Prophylaxis. Genetic counseling is required for families of patients with Huntington's Chorea; during the meetings it is necessary to explain the risk of occurrence of the disease in a future offspring.

2. Hepatolenticular Degeneration.

A chronic progressive inherited degenerative disease characterized by concurrent
damage to the subcortical ganglia and the liver.

Synonyms. Hepatocerebral dystrophy, Wilson-Konovalov disease.

Frequency. The disorder is rare but encountered all around the world. According to some investigators the frequency of the homozygous state is 1:200 000 /5, 8/.

Etiology and pathogenesis. The disorder is inherited in autosomal dominant pattern. With the aid of DNA-recombination method evidence has been obtained for the localization of the pathologic gene in chromosome 13 /12/. Genetically induced impairment of the synthesis of the protein ceruloplasmin, which is one of the α-2 globulins transporting copper, is most important in the pathogenesis. A result of this is high concentration of copper in the blood followed by copper deposition in a number of organs, mainly the liver, brain, cornea, kidneys, etc. The toxic effect of copper is associated with blocking of sulfhydrile groups in the oxidation ferments which leads to impairment of oxidation recovery processes in the cells. When determining catecholamines, increased excretion of dopamine is found in these patients, which is related to the development of extrapyramidal motor disturbances.

Pathomorphology. Degenerative lesions are observed in the brain, liver, spleen, kidneys and vitreous body. Dystrophic changes in neurons are also found with focal liquification, microcyst formation and glial expansion. Small hemorrhages and perivascular edema is seen among small cerebral vessels. Hepatic lesions are in the form of macronodular cirrhosis or mixed cirrhosis. The green corneal ring of Kaiser-Fleischer is observed as a result of copper deposition in the cornea. It is pathognomonic for the disease.

Clinical manifestations. It is polymorphous and is determined by the coexistence of symptoms of damage to the nervous system and some internal organs, mainly the liver. Several clinical variants are distinguished depending on the prevalent symptom complex:

- abdominal form: its course is characterized by severe hepatic impairment with icterus, hepatosplenomegaly, ascites, fever with concurrent hemorrhages, gastrointestinal disturbances. Patients soon die of hepatic failure, even before cirrhosis and neurologic symptoms develop. Endocrine disorders are also frequently encountered: infantile stature, very high stature, menstrual disturbances, etc.;

- early rigid-arrhythmohyperkinetic form: It is characterized by rapid development of general rigidity and arrhythmic athetosic or torsion dystonic hyperkinesias. Rigidity affects all muscles of the trunk, extremities, chewing, swallowing and speech systems. Amimia, dysphagia and dysarthria are observed. The gait becomes stiff hopping. Retro-, antero- and lateropulsion are discovered. Muscle rigidity can increase paroxysmally with some movements and especially with emotions. Patients frequently remain in unusual postures. Contractures often develop in distal parts of the extremities and leave patients completely handicapped. This form usually begins from 7 to 15 years of age and visceral disturbances can occur at 3-5 years of age; hepatic impairment is the prevalent one and it usually precedes the neurologic problems;

- tremor form: It begins at a later age between 20 and 35 years of age and follows a benign course. Hepatic dysfunction is slightly pronounced. In this case rigidity does not occur and there is a characteristic tremor in the extremities which can involve the whole body. Patients have a flapping tremor. Tremor may involve facial muscles, speech muscles and even eye muscles. Speech becomes scanned. Tremor of the soft palate, vocal cords, respiratory muscles and diaphragm is sometimes seen. Cerebellar symptoms are usually present also;

- shivering-rigid form: It presents as combination of symptoms from the rigid and tremor forms. Tremor in this form of the disease is more expressed in the arms and rigidity is more expressed in the legs. Neurologic symptoms develop at approximately 15-20 years of age;

- extrapyramidal-cortical form: This form differs from the others in the more severe damage to the cerebral cortex. In these cases pyramidal mono- and hemipareses develop along with extrapyramidal pathology. Jacksonian or generalized epileptic seizures are frequently observed. Intellect declines, severe personality degradation occurs, emotional-volutional sphere and mental activity change.

Diagnosis and differential diagnosis. The family history data, the characteristic clinical manifestations, the green ring of Kaiser-Fleischer and the biochemical tests demonstrating a low blood level of ceruloplasmin, as well as the increased excretion of copper with the urine confirm the diagnosis /89/. The reference range for ceruloplasmin is 240-450 mg/l and in hepatocerebral dystrophy it decreases to 0-200 mg/l. there is also increased urinary excretion of copper exceeding 160 μmol/l, the reference range being 14.22-22.6 μmol/l; and hyperaminoaciduria exceeding 7.1-14.3 mmol/24 hours, the reference range being up to 7.1 mmol/24 hours. With the aid of needle biopsy copper content in the liver is established, which is extremely elevated, 500-3 000 μg/g dry weight, the mean reference being 32 μg/g.

Differential diagnosis should be made with Huntington's Chorea /its akinetic-rigid variant/, with cerebellar ataxias /in which there is flapping tremor/, with Minor's essential tremor /in the early stage/ and with Hallervorden-Spatz disease /in it the metabolism of iron and catecholamines is disturbed, it is inherited in autosomal recessive pattern/. It is also necessary to differentiate the disease from postencephalic Parkinsonism, disseminated sclerosis /Bauer's criteria are used for its diagnosis/, some forms of neuroses in which flapping tremor is observed, etc.

Evolution. The course is progressive and is not significantly influenced by therapeutic measures. The average life expectancy for the patients is approximately 6 years.

Treatment. Pathogenic treatment is based on administering drugs facilitating copper excretion from the organism, mainly D-Penicillamine /Cuprenil/ or Unitiol. D-Penicillamine is administered at a dose of 0.15 g/day for 2-3 months and after that the dose is gradually increased to 6-10 tablets of 0.15 mg/day. Treatment continues throughout the patient's life. If this drug is not well tolerated by the patients, Unitiol is administered at a dose of 5 ml/day of the 5% solution intramuscularly in one-month or two-month treatment courses with a respite from treatment for 2-3 months. In case of pronounced hyperkinesias agents like L-DOPA, Sinemet, etc. can be added. The patients' food must contain less honey and be rich in carbohydrates and vitamins.

Prophylaxis. Genetic counseling. Giving birth again is not recommended in cases of an affected child in the family.

3. Parkinson Disease.

A chronic progressive disease, characterized by akinetic-rigid syndrome and typical tremor, which result from damage mainly of substantia nigra and globus pallidus.

Frequency. The disorder is frequent in all geographic areas but there is no precise data about the morbidity. It is known that approximately 5% of elderly people suffer from Parkinsonism / Parkinson's syndrome/ which develops due to another main disease in contrast to Parkinson's Disease.

Etiology and pathogenesis. Not well understood. It is considered that coexistence of familial hereditary predisposition and effect of exogenous factors is required for the development of Parkinson's Disease. Endocrine dysfunction, which appears with age, is one of the predisposing factors. There are families with clusters of cases with clinical manifestations of the "pure" syndrome which is inherited in autosomal dominant pattern and presents at an earlier age. Concordance is found in these cases: approximately 6% in mono- and polyzygotes. There exists the so-called Guam variant of Parkinson-dementia complex which is autosomal dominant and of high incidence. These data suggest that most probably exogenous /mainly toxic/ factors add to p genetic redisposition /autosomal dominant/, and genetic factors determine the susceptibility of the nervous system /16/.

Symptomatic Parkinsonism develops quite frequently in central nervous infections: following primary lethargic encephalitis or other viral encephalitis, in encephalitis, caused by various nonviral infectious agents such as tuberculosis, malaria, rheumatic fever, etc. Very often Parkinsonism is also manifested in vascular disorders of the nervous system: cerebral atherosclerosis, hypertension, following brain insults. Some industrial intoxications with manganese, lead-carbon dioxide, etc. lead to the development of so-called toxic Parkinsonism. In case of overdose of some drugs /reserpine derivatives, phenothiazines, Methyldopa, etc./ drug-induced Parkinsonism occurs. More rarely the disorder is observed in central nervous system traumas, tumors, metabolic disturbances, etc. /21/.

The leading pathogenic mechanism of the disease is a result of the disturbed metabolism of catecholamines /dopamine, acetylcholine, noradrenalin/ in the extrapyramidal system. Dopamine possesses an independent mediator function in movement realization. Under normal conditions its concentration in basal ganglia significantly exceeds its amount in other structures of the nervous system. Acetylcholine is a mediator of excitation in substantia nigra, globus pallidus and nucleus caudatus. Dopamine and acetylcholine are antagonistic; dopamine has an inhibition activity. In case of injury to substantia nigra and globus pallidus the concentration of dopamine in nucleus caudatus decreases, the dopamine-acetylcholine steady state is disturbed and the function of the extrapyramidal system is impaired. Under normal conditions impulses are modulated in direction of inhibition of nucleus caudatus and substantia nigra and activation of globus pallidus. Suspension of the functions of substantia nigra results in a blockage of the impulses coming from the extrapyramidal cortex and putamen to the anterior spinal horns. Meanwhile pathologic impulses originating from pallidum and substantia nigra reach anterior root cells As a result impulse circulation in the system of α- and γ-motoneurons of the spinal cord is increased with prevalence of α-activity, which leads to development of pallido-nigral rigidity of muscle fibers and tremor: the cardinal signs of Parkinsonism.

Pathomorphology. Degenerative lesions are found in all melanin-containing cells of the brain stem. Substantia nigra and globus pallidus are most severely affected, but nucleus caudatus, thalamus opticus, hypothalamus and locus ceruleus are also damaged. Dopamine-containig cells in substantia nigra are most severely affected which leads to degeneration of nigro-strial dopaminergic pathways, acute decline in dopamine synthesis and secretion in the striatum /81/. In dopaminergic neurons inclusions are found: the so-called Lewy bodies, but they are not specific markers of Parkinson's Disease /34/.

Clinical manifestations. The disorder is characterized by three cardinal signs: akinesia, rigidity and tremor /26/. Autonomic dysfunction and mental changes are frequent. Akinetic- rigid syndrome is demonstrated with plastic rigidity as "Negro's cogwheel rigidity", poor and slowed movements, absence of physiological synkinesias. The patient's posture and gait change: the body is leaned forward, the arms are semiflexed in the elbows and held tight to the trunk. Patients walk with small irregular steps and have difficulties with lifting their feet off the floor. During movement their legs are flexed in the knees, physiological dyskinesias in the arms disappear: the so-called acheirokinesia. Pulsion symptoms – propulsion, antero-pulsion and latero-pulsion – are often observed. The patients' face is with masked expression, the speech is quiet and monotonic. The hand-writing is minute, uneven: micrography. In some patients with severe akinesia sudden rapid movements are sometimes seen: running, climbing stairs, etc. Complete lack of movement develops later. Static tremor is also very typical of Parkinsonism. It mainly affects distal parts of the extremities, often resembles counting money, etc. with disease progression the tremor also affects other parts of the extremities, the face, the tongue, the head and the soft palate. The tremor is rhythmic with a frequency of 4-6 movements/second, of various amplitude. It is more pronounced in the arms than in the legs and decreases with movement. During the late stages of the disease the tremor becomes permanent. Hyperkinesias increase with emotional stress, tiredness, and decrease with rest, and disappear during sleep. Autonomic dysfunction is frequent: excessive salivation and sweating, "oily face", vasomotor fluctuations, tachycardia, acrocyanosis, subfebrile temperature and trophic skin changes. As a rule tendon reflexes are not altered. In atherosclerotic and postencephalic Parkinsonism, however, they can be pathologically increased, along with the presence of other pyramidal symptoms. In postencephalic Parkinsonism the gaze is sometimes fixated upwards with the head turned aside, and this can persist for several minutes to several hours. These crises can coexist with disturbances of accommodation and convergence. Mental changes are characterized by bradyphrenia, emotional disorders / lowered initiativeness, emotional lability, sometimes irritability, hypochondrias/. Dementia gradually develops. 3 major forms of Parkinsonism are distinguished based on the clinical course: tremor, tremor-rigid and rigid-bradykinetic. The presence of almost constant tremor movements of middle or large amplitude affecting the extremities, the tongue, the head and the mandible is characteristic for the tremor form. This form is most frequent in postencephalic and posttraumatic Parkinsonism. The tremor-rigid form is characterized by tremor, localized in distal parts of the extremities with concurrent muscle rigidity. The rigid-bradykinetic form of Parkinsonism goes with plastic rigidity, progressive slowing of movements to complete invalidization, development of muscle contractures and flexion posture of the patient. This form is observed most frequently in atherosclerotic Parkinsonism and follows the most unfavorable course.

Diagnosis and differential diagnosis. First Parkinson's Disease must be differentiated from Parkinson's syndrome. Eye movement disorders are characteristic of postencephalic Parkinsonism; furthermore torticollis, focal manifestations of torsion dystonia, etc. can be observed, which are never present in the other forms. Sleep disorders, respiratory disturbances, autonomic paroxysms, etc. are encountered. Posttraumatic Parkinsonism predominantly affects middle and young aged people. It develops after serious cerebral traumas. Pulsion phenomena, respiratory and swallowing difficulties, cataplexy are rare in this form. Vestibular dysfunction, memory and intellectual deficit, visual hallucinations / due to cortical lesions/ are frequent. In Parkinsonism, resulting from lead, mercury, etc. intoxication professional history is important, as well as isolation of the toxic substances from urine and CSF. Drug-induced Parkinsonism recovers following discontinuation of the respective drug /Reserpine, phenothiazines, etc./. In atherosclerotic Parkinsonism tremor and rigidity are combined with signs of cerebral atherosclerosis or develop following acute disturbances of cerebral blood flow. Focal neurologic manifestations appear with pyramidal and pseudobulbar symptoms. Blood lipid levels are increased. Reoencephalographic investigation demonstrates flattening of the curve, which assumes the form of a "plateau", and Doppler sonography discovers atherosclerotic changes in the examined cerebral vessels. Senile atherosclerotic dementia must be distinguished; in it severe mental disorders and feeble-mindedness develop. In the differential diagnostic plan one should also consider progressive supranuclear ophthalmoplegia /Steele-Richardson-Olszewski syndrome/. This is a dystrophic process of unknown etiology, with neuronal loss, demielinization and gliosis, affecting mainly the mesencephalon, pallidum and white matter. An onset at approximately 50-60 years of age, presence of vertical gaze paralysis, extrapyramidal rigidity and dementia are characteristic clinical manifestations.

Manifestations of Parkinsonism can be observed in Fridreich's disease, olivopontocerebellar atrophy, Creutzfeldt-Jacob Disease, etc. Cerebellar ataxia is noted in these disorders along with the akinetic-rigid syndrome.

Evolution. The prognosis of Parkinsonism is unfavorable. It depends on the etiology, the disease form and the therapeutic response of the patients. Postencephalic Parkinsonism has the longest life-expectancy /approximately 15-20 years/, and atherosclerotic Parkinsonism has the shortest one /3-5 years/. Death occurs due to decubital complications, pneumonias and urinary tract infections, which respond poorly to treatment.

Treatment. It is described in details in the general neurology course. Drugs that are already recognized are used: anticholinesterase agents /Parkisan, Norakin, Akineton, etc./, dopaminergic /L-DOPA, inhibitors of DOPA-carboxylase and combination of the two agents, Sinemet, Madopar/, dopamine agonists /Parlodel, Viregyt, etc./.

Prophylaxis. Because hereditary forms are relatively rare prophylaxis is directed mainly towards early diagnostics and timely treatment of the main diseases leading to development of Parkinson's syndrome.

4. Torsion Dystonia.

A chronic progressive hereditary disorder of the extrapyramidal system characterized by peculiar changes in muscle tone, leading to awkward posturing of the body and slow, tonic hyperkinesias.

Synonyms. Deforming muscular dystonia, Ziehen-Oppenheim Disease.

Etiology and pathogenesis. There is idiopathic /familial/ torsion dystonia and symptomatic which can develop in other disturbances of the extrapyramidal system, e.g. epidemic encephalitis, cerebral palsy, tumors, hepatocerebral dystrophy, Huntington's Chorea, etc.

Idiopathic /familial/ dystonia can be inherited both in autosomal dominant and autosomal recessive pattern, and recessive inheritance is related to more severe course of the disease. The primary genetic biochemical defect of the disease has not been discovered yet.

The change in the functional activity of the extrapyramidal neurotransmitter systems /dopaminergic systems, the systems of serotonin and norepinephrine/ is considered to be of great importance in the pathogenesis of torsion dystonia; this is the reason for the impaired central regulation of muscle tone. As a result of this reciprocal innervation mechanisms are impaired, pathologic "contraction of antagonists" develops, which in turn leads to development of peculiar hyperkinesias and abnormal posturing of the body /10/.

Pathomorphology. Degenerative lesions are found in the brain, mainly in the area of the basal ganglia /nucleus caudatus, globus pallidus/, nucleus ruber, nucleus dentatus of the cerebellum. Glia develops in place of dead neurons.

Clinical manifestations. The onset of the disease is during childhood or adolescence, between 5 and 15 years of age, and more rarely /with dominant inheritance/ later, between 25 and 40 years of age.

Torsion dystonia is characterized by marked clinical polymorphism. Significant variability in the expressivity of the pathologic gene is observed, even among one family's members. There are two forms of the disease: generalized and localized.

The generalized form is characterized by severely pronounced tonic hyperkinesias affecting the muscles of the trunk, neck and extremities. As a result of these hyperkinesias, the body becomes distorted in different directions. Not infrequently the spinal column shows pathologic lordoses. The patient's head is tilted backwards /retrocollis/, leans to one side or forward /antecollis/, the extremities assume unusual, awkward positions. Deformations and contractures of joints develop gradually. Hyperkinesias are intensified with random movements and especially walking, and decreased in lying position and during sleep. Muscle tone changes are characterized by coexistence of extrapyramidal rigidity and hypotonia and depend on the body's posture at the given moment. Muscle rigidity develops in the advanced stages of the disease. Disturbances in swallowing, breathing and speech can develop with involvement of the facial, swallowing and intercostal muscles.

The localized form of torsion dystonia, which is more frequent, is characterized by muscle tone changes and hyperkinesias, affecting only separate muscle groups of the trunk and extremities. Rigidity also affects only separate muscles and may lead to improper position of the foot and disturbed gait. Cramps during writing may develop when hand muscles are affected. Other variants of the localized form of torsion dystonia are: spastic torticollis /in it tonic hyperkinesias in cervical muscles lead to wry neck and forceful turning of the head/, oromandibular dystonia, blepharospasm, dysphonia, Rulph's intention tremor /occurring more often in the lower extremities at the beginning of active movement/, etc.

Diagnosis and differential diagnosis. The diagnosis is made on the basis of the characteristic for the disease tone alterations and hyperkinesias, the early onset of the disease and positive family history. The differential diagnosis of torsion dystonia must first be made with symptomatic forms of the disorder. Exogenously induced phenocopies of the disease are distinguished by their nonprogressive course, marked asymmetry of the pathologic changes, presence of other /except extrapyramidal/ symptoms arising from the nervous system. Torsion dystonia is differentiated from hepatocerebral dystrophy /mostly from the early rigid-arrhythmohyperkinetic form/ by the lack of hepatic dysfunction, the absence of the green corneal ring of Kaiser-Fleischer, as well as the normal serum levels of copper. Torsion dystonia is distinguished from double athetosis by its progressive course, later onset of the disease /double athetosis begins during the first few months of life/, the localization of the hyperkinesias /in double athetosis they affect manly the distal parts of the extremities/. Furthermore double athetosis is not hereditary and in it there are no pyramidal signs, pathologically increased reflexes, pathologic reflexes from the Babinski group, etc. Parkinson's Disease should also be considered. However it affects older people, and besides hyperkinesias and tone alterations there are other symptoms, characteristic of Parkinsonism only. In torsion dystonia intellect is generally preserved, the mental or autonomic problems, characteristic of Parkinson's Disease, are not present.

Evolution. The symptoms of torsion dystonia progress incessantly. Sometimes there are remissions of variable duration. Gradually invalidization and death occur, especially in the generalized form.

Treatment. When extrapyramidal muscle rigidity predominates in the clinical course, drugs with L-DOPA as an active ingredient /Madopar, etc./ are administered with gradual increase in the dose. Their average daily dose is 200-500 mg. the drugs are administered for a long period. In case of reduced efficacy or side effects /secondary akinesias or myoclonic or choreic hyperkinesias, hypotension and arrhythmia/, dopaminergic agents are added: dopamine agonists, MAO inhibitors, etc. If hyperkinesias occur, benzodiazepines are used: Antelepsin, Chlordiazepoxide, etc.

In the hyperkinetic form of torsion dystonia, in contrast to the first case, drugs inhibiting the dopaminergic systems are applied. Phenothiazines and buthyrophenone agents are used: Stelazine, Haloperidol, etc., which block dopamine receptors. This effect is enhanced by adding benzodiazepine derivatives.

Administration of agonists of D2 dopamine receptors /e.g. Parlodel/, which are D1 receptor antagonists simultaneously, has a beneficial effect on torsion dystonic motor disturbances, including spastic torticollis. General supportive and stimulating agents are also used: Nootropil, Encephabol, Cerebrolysin. Physiotherapeutic and orthopedic procedures, directed at improving muscle hypertonia, are also carried out. In some cases surgical treatment is applied: destruction of the ventrolateral nucleus of the thalamus, which when performed unilaterally can lead to reduction or even disappearance of the torsion dystonic hyperkinesias on the contralateral half of the body. In extremely severe cases the operation is done bilaterally.

Prophylaxis. Genetic counseling. The recessive form of the disease is particularly hazardous. In such cases no more childbirths in the family should be allowed.

5. Familial Tremor.

A hereditary disorder which main clinical manifestation is tremor, localized in the arms, neck and head.

Synonyms. Tremophilia, Minor's essential familial tremor, hereditary tremor, névrose trémolante.

Frequency. It shows significant variation in the individual populations studied: from 4 to 55/1000 people in the age group over 40 years.

Etiology and pathogenesis. The disease is transmitted in autosomal dominant pattern with variable expressivity of the pathologic gene. This expressivity may vary significantly both among different families and among different members of one family. Sporadic cases are also encountered. The disbalance between adrenergic and cholinergic systems lies in the basis of the pathogenesis of the disease. The adrenergic system is activated, which is accompanied by excitation of β-adrenoreceptors and inhibition of the cholinergic and serotoninergic systems /46, 73/.

Pathomorphology. In most cases no pathologic changes are found in the brain. Sometimes discrete degenerative lesions in the striatum are seen.

Clinical manifestations. The disease may begin at any age including childhood and adolescence. Nevertheless middle-aged and elderly patients predominate. A great variety regarding age has been noted in different families. The main clinical manifestation is tremor with a frequency of 4-6-11 Hz which is postural in nature and does not increase with motion. Tremor is absent at rest to the contrary of Parkinson's Disease. Trembling is most often localized in the fingers and wrists, also affecting the muscles of the neck and head. Sometimes the head moves forward-backward or side-to-side as if the patient is saying "yes" or "no". isolated tremor of the arms and/or head is the only manifestation of the disease for a long time. Sometimes cramps while writing or spastic torticollis is observed. With disease progression tremor affects also parts of the trunk, pharyngeal muscles, the vocal cords, and more infrequently the lower extremities. Tremor frequency decreases and its amplitude increases with age. Essential tremor is enhanced by stress, emotional and physical efforts, nicotine use, coffee, etc. tremor is usually more intense in the morning. It decreases when the patient's attention is distracted and with alcohol use, and disappears during sleep. In rare instances stiff gait, muscle rigidity in the lower extremities and discrete cerebellar symptomatics can be observed. It is noted that if the disease begins at an early age, the tremor most often appears in the arms. In some cases patients are forced to change their profession and in other work capacity is maintained for a long time.

Diagnosis and differential diagnosis. Usually the diagnosis does not present a difficulty. The characteristic tremor, positive family history, genealogic and biochemical investigations make it easier. As a differential diagnosis one should consider physiological tremor, intensified in situations of stress, some endocrine disorders /thyrotoxicosis/, some intoxications /with alcohol, mercury, lead, neuroleptics/. Moreover tremor may be a sign of another degenerative disease /Parkinsonism, hepatocerebral dystrophy, torsion dystonia, cerebellar ataxias/. In these cases the tremor has different characteristics, there are also a number of other symptoms.

Evolution. As a rule the disease course is slow and progressive. In general the prognosis is relatively favorable and work capacity is maintained for a long time. The course of the disease is more unfavorable in homozygous carriers of the pathologic gene whose parents are both affected.

Treatment. B-blockers – Propranolol, Obsidan, etc. - are most effective, with an average daily dose of approximately 120 mg. Benzodiazepines – Antelepsin, Diazepam - also exhibit a good effect. Phenobarbital is used at a dose of 1-1.5 mg/kg. Anticholinergic agents – Norakin, etc. - are prescribed in the usual doses. If there is no beneficial response to conservative therapy, stereoataxic surgical operations of the basal ganglia and especially of some areas of the thalamus are done.

Prophylaxis. Genetic counseling. Childbearing is not recommended in cases of two affected potential parents.

6. Fahr's Syndrome.

A symptom complex which results from "idiopathic" non-atherosclerotic calcification of intracerebral vessels in the striopallidal area.

Synonyms. Cerebral calculosis. Idiopathic non-atherosclerotic calcification of intracerebral vessels.

Etiology and pathogenesis. The etiology is unknown. There are also familial cases which are probably inherited in autosomal recessive pattern. Disturbances in calcium and phosphorus metabolism are considered to play a role in the pathogenesis, and possibly hyperphosphatemia is of great importance. The blood levels of calcium and phosphorus, however, are usually within normal limits.

Pathomorphology. Calcification of intracerebral vessels in pallidum, putamen, thalamus, substantia nigra, nucleus ruber, etc. is found. Degenerative changes develop in brain tissue /6/.

Clinical manifestations. The classic idiopathic form can be asymptomatic or with polymorphic clinical manifestations including various epileptic seizures, extrapyramidal symptoms / mainly hyperkinesias/, sometimes pyramidal signs as well, slowly progressing moderate dementia, etc. Another form is also described, in which dysfunction of the parathyroid glands is established, resulting in disturbances of the calcium-phosphorus metabolism / hyperparathyroidism, hypoparathyroidism/.

Diagnosis and differential diagnosis. Symmetric calcifications of intracerebral vessels in basal ganglia are seen on craniograms and rarely on CT. as a differential diagnosis one should consider a large number of diseases which also demonstrate intracranial calcifications: aneurisms and arterio-venous malformations, hematomas, craniopharyngioma, cysticercosis, toxoplasmosis, neurolues, tuberous sclerosis, Alzheimer's Disease, Pick's Disease, Hallervorden-Spatz Disease, etc.

Evolution. The course is slow, progressing over a few years, but precise life-expectancy has not been established yet.

Treatment. Symptomatic.

Prophylaxis. Timely diagnostics of the classic idiopathic form and its differentiation from the symptomatic forms with the aid of roentgenograms and CT.

7. Hallervorden-Spatz Syndrome.

A degenerative disorder characterized by progressive extrapyramidal rigidity, akinesia, hyperkinesias and dementia.

Synonyms. Progressive degeneration of pallidum. Pigmentary degenerative syndrome of pallidum.

Etiology and pathogenesis. Not known. It is thought to be inherited in autosomal recessive pattern, but there are also sporadic cases.

Pathomorphology. Spheroid bodies are found in basal ganglia and nerve endings, in which there is significant deposition of green-brown pigment containing iron. Large amount of iron is also deposited in the cortex and in the cerebellum. Furthermore, diffuse changes in neurons are observed, mostly in the basal ganglia and cortex, glial cells with large nuclei are seen, which resemble the alterations in Alzheimer's Disease. Sometimes pigmentary retinopathy develops.

Clinical manifestations. The first symptoms develop around 10 years of age. The primary manifestation of the disease is progressive extrapyramidal rigidity. Along with it choreoathetosic or torsion dystonic hyperkinesias are observed, as well as pathologic curvature of the legs leading to joint deformation and tremor, similar to the Parkinsonian one. Progressive dementia is noted in most patients, frequently combined with emotional disturbances. Sometimes however in some families patients' speech and mental state are not altered. In other cases coexistence of extrapyramidal symptoms with pyramidal signs and hyperpigmentation of the skin is found. Visual disturbances are discovered, which are due to retinal pigment degeneration and optic nerve atrophy.

Diagnosis and differential diagnosis. When establishing the diagnosis besides the characteristic extrapyramidal symptoms and dementia manifestations, performing CT and MRI is of great importance; they find hydrocephalus and diffuse cerebral atrophy, mainly in the brain stem and the cerebellum, and it is also confirmed by the morphological changes in dead patients. Differential diagnosis should be made first with hepatocerebral dystrophy in which there is disturbed metabolism of copper, hepatic cirrhosis and a corneal ring of Kaiser-Fleischer. Pallidal degeneration also presents serious difficulties. In it globus pallidus is predominantly affected; it begins between 10 and 30 years of age, and the cardinal clinical manifestation is tremor, pseudobulbar symptoms may be added in late stages.

Evolution. The disorder follows a chronic progressive course. Patients die of intercurrent infections within 10-20 years.

Treatment. Temporary amelioration of the symptoms is achieved by administering L-DOPA and cholinolytic agents.

Prophylaxis. Genetic counseling.

8. Tourette's Syndrome.

Multiple tics, including vocal ones, together with myoclonus-like hyperkinesias, coprolalia, copropraxia, mannerism and awkward grimaces.

Synonyms. Tourette's Disease, Gilles de la Tourette's Disease, Brissaud's variable chorea, myoplasia impulssiva, convulsive tic disease /maladie des tics convulsifs/, mimic convulsion neurosis / mimische krampneurose/, koordinitierte erinnerrungskraempfe, tic disease, generalized tic, impulsive myospasia.

Frequency. The disorder is rare but nevertheless its frequency is considered to be approximately 5/1 000 000 people. According to some authors the incidence of the disease is much higher /0.03% in the US/ and the male to female ratio is 3:1.

Etiology and pathogenesis. The etiology of the disorder is unknown. In one third of the cases a family relationship between the patients is discovered. Autososmal dominant pattern of inheritance is supposed but there is no evidence for it. In other cases authors assume that there is influence of infections, intoxications and traumas during the prenatal period of development. Disturbed balance in mediator systems of striatum with prevalence of the nigro-striatic dopaminergic system probably lies in the basis of the pathogenensis.

Pathomorphology. The disorder is not studied in details due to its benign course and results from the autopsies of the few autopsied patients are contradictory. In several cases degenerative changes of the neurons in nucleus caudatus and globus pallidus are described with no proliferation of glia.

Clinical manifestations. The disorder begins in childhood, around the 10th year, but sometimes earlier. Tic-like hyperkinesias of facial muscles appear first: blinking, trembling of mimic muscles, opening of the mouth opening and sticking the tongue out, lip bulging. With disease progression tics involve muscles of the neck, shoulder girdle, trunk and extremities. Gradually sound symptoms are added /vocal tics/: coughing, barking, whistling, pronouncing separate words, whispering, etc. Coprolalia appears /utterance of obscene words/. Coprolalia occurs with no reason whatsoever, and curses are loud and sharp, often with improper pronunciation. Copropraxia /obscene gestures/ is also encountered as an equivalent to swearing. Echo-symptoms /echolalia and echopraxia/ are observed in many patients. Children's behavior is affected, reactive depression with irritability and aggression manifestations appears, which can alternate with periods of lively and cheerful behavior /51/.

Diagnosis and differential diagnosis. Along with tic hyperkinesias, which are observed with other degenerative disorders as well, coprolalia and copropraxia are specific for Gilles de la Tourette's symptom and are not encountered elsewhere. Biochemical tests in this syndrome sometimes demonstrate decreased level of homovanillic acid and 5-hydroxyindol-ylacetic acid. This indirectly suggests reduced concentration of dopamine and 5-hydroxytriptamine in patients' brains. Neurologic examination and EEG did not show specific changes in patients. Differential diagnosis is made with Sydenham's chorea /in it there is rheumatism etiology, cardiac changes/, with Huntington's Chorea, with transient tics, schizophrenia, neuroses and psychoses. In some cases the differentiation of Tourette's Disease from Lesch-Nyhan's Syndrome is interesting; the latter can also include coprolalia. In it, however, the onset is much earlier, the intellect is severely affected and the inheritance is autosomal recessive.

Evolution. The course of the disorder is slow and favorable regarding patient's life. Tics and other symptoms tend to increase progressively and make patient's everyday life difficult.

Treatment. Agents from the benzodiazepine group - Diazepam and Clonazepam – have a tranquilizing effect and are frequently administered to patients. A beneficial response to the usage of the α-adrenoreceptic agonist Clophilin at a dose of 0.125-0.3 mg/day is achieved in approximately 50% of patients, probably due to its influence over central noradrenergic structures. Haloperidol is administered at a dose of 0.25-0.5 mg/day, with a gradual increase of the dose. Antidepressants and psychotherapy are applied with some effect.

Prophylaxis. Because of the unknown pattern of inheritance of the disorder and the unknown etiology, there are no effective prophylactic measures.

Chapter III

HEREDITARY ATAXIAS

Primary dystrophic diseases affecting cerebellar structures, with various pattern of inheritance and significant clinical polymorphism of multiform nosological units and syndromes. These diseases are classified according to topics, and two groups are arbitrarily differentiated: spinocerebellar dystrophies and cerebellar dystrophies.

1. Spinocerebellar Atrophies.

1.1 Friedreich's Disease.
A chronic progressive disorder, the major clinical manifestation of which is spinal
ataxia.

Synonyms. Friedreich's hereditary ataxia. Spinal ataxia.

Frequency. This is the most prevalent heredoataxia. The median frequency of hereditary ataxias being 2-4/1 000 000 people, Friedreich's Disease accounts for about 55% of this group of diseases. Men and women are equally affected.

Etiology and pathogenesis. The disorder is hereditary and is transmitted in autosomal recessive pattern with reduced penetrance of the pathologic gene. Consanguinity is noted to be of higher frequency among patients' parents. Sporadic cases of the disease are also described. Dysfunction of the spinal systems for motion coordination and mainly of the dorsal columns is considered to lie in the basis of the pathogenesis; and it is assumed that impaired oxidation of lactate dehydrogenase and reduced synthesis of acetylcholine in the brain stem, the cerebellum, afferent and efferent spinal systems, play a certain role /42, 69/.

Pathomorphology. Degeneration of the dorsal and lateral columns of the spinal cord is particularly characteristic of the disease. Goll's collumn is affected more severely than Burdach's column. Cells of Clarke's column and spinocerebellar tracts originating from it are also affected. Damage to pyramidal tracts usually starts from the lumbar region of the spinal cord. Degenerative changes are also found in Purkinje cells and brain stem nuclei. Peripheral nerves are also affected.

Clinical manifestations. The disease begins between 7 and 15 years of age. The main symptom is spinocerebellar ataxia. Cerebellar symptoms come predominantly from the vermis. The gait is very ataxic. Patients walk with a broad-based gait, staggering from side to side. It was described by Scharcot as tabetic-cerebellar. Spastic ataxia is also observed. Romberg's sign is positive. In the beginning the movements of the arms are slightly affected but with disease progression their coordination is impaired and hand-writing changes. Patients' facial expression changes, the speech becomes slow, nonmodulated, dysarthric. Dysmetria, adiadochokinesia and various hyperkinesias, which generally accompany active movements, may appear. Muscle tone is decreased. In late stages low spastic paraparesis may develop, as well as tremor of the hands and head, visual and hearing impairment. Cognitive disorders are also observed /40/.

A number of somatic disorders are characteristic for Friedreich's Disease: mostly skeletal abnormalities and cardiac involvement. Kyphoscoliosis and a typical foot deformity /high arches, flexion of the toes, mainly of the I[st] one in the proximal phalanx, joint deformity/, the so-called Friedreich's foot. Cardiac involvement includes tachycardia, paroxysmal stenocardia attacks, shortness of breath during physical effort, cardiomegaly and systolic murmurs. ECG shows rhythm and conduction abnormalities, T-wave inversion, P-wave deformity. Congenital heart disease is often present. In a number of cases Friedreich's Ataxia is coexistent with Diabetes Mellitus. Other endocrine disorders, that are noted, are infantilism and hypogonadism. Congenital cataract is rarer. Anomalies vary from family to family. They are assumed to be a manifestation of the heterozygous carrier state of the pathologic gene. Sometimes such features are the first manifestation of the disease in childhood.

Neurologic examination finds pronounced nystagmus, ataxia in the arms and legs, dysmetria, adiadochokinesia, scanned speech, disturbed position and vibration sense. An early symptom is decrease or absence of tendon and periostal reflexes. The combination of positive Babinski sign with knee- and Achilles- areflexia and muscle hypotonia is typical. First tendon and periostal reflexes disappear in the lower extremities, and later areflexia spreads to arms /52, 64/. Otoneurologic examination demonstrates vestibular disturbances and hearing is often impaired. Atrophy of the optic nerves and the nerves controlling eye movements is not frequently observed but changes in visual evoked responses are almost always discovered. Mental state is usually preserved, but it is often affected in later stages of the disease. EEG shows disturbed α- and β-rhythm, presence of irregular sharp waves and groups of slow waves.

Diagnosis and differential diagnosis. The disorder is distinguished by the characteristic atactic manifestations combined with "Fridreich's" foot, spinal column deformities, cardiac and endocrine abnormalities. As a differential diagnosis one should have in mind multiple sclerosis, cerebral syphilis, funicular myelosis, cerebellar and olivo-ponto-cerebellar degeneration, etc /91/. Cases with atypical Friedreich's Disease present a particular challenge: symptoms characteristic of cerebellar ataxias, familial spastic paraplegia, neural muscular atrophy, appear along with ataxia. Hereditary areflexic dystasia /Roussy-Levy syndrome/ is of special interest: in the past it was considered to be a form of Friedreich's Disease, and today prevails the believe that it is a phenotypic variant of neural muscular atrophy. CT plays a certain role in differentiating of cerebellar ataxias: it shows cerebellar atrophy.

Ataxia may be combined with pyramidal symptoms in disseminated sclerosis. The latter differs from Friedreich's Disease in its later onset, remitting course, multifocal symptomatics, temporal paleness of papillae, CSF changes and negative family history.

Evolution. The disorder progresses slowly. Patients live for 10-15 years after the appearance of the first symptoms.

Treatment. Symptomatic. Special rehabilitation procedures are used, aimed at improving coordination disturbances. Vitamins, nootropic medications /Nootropil, Aminalon, Cerebrolysin/, cardiotonics are applied, and in some cases orthopedic corrections of the deformities /78/.

Prophylaxis. Genetic counseling.

2.Cerebellar Atrophies. Forms and Symptoms.
2.1. Pierre-Mari's Hereditary Cerebellar Ataxia.

A chronic progressive disorder the cardinal feature of which is cerebellar ataxia.

Synonyms. Pierre-Marie-Sanger-Brown's disease, Nonne-Pierre-Marie's syndrome, cerebellar heredoataxia, hereditary cerebellar ataxia, hereditary cerebellar ataxia with spasticity.

Etiology and pathogenesis. The disorder is hereditary and is transmitted in autosomal dominant pattern. The pathologic gene has high penetrance and development of the disease is seen in almost all generations.

Pathomorphology. The major pathoanatomic substrate of the disease is cerebellar hypoplasia along with atrophy of inferior olives, pons and cerebral cortex. Degeneration of the spinal systems is found as well as involvement of the optic and other cranial nerves.

Clinical manifestations. The main clinical sign is ataxia which resembles the one in Friedreich's Disease. The disorder usually begins with gait disturbances, to which ataxia of the arms, affected speech and facial expression are added. Static ataxia is pronounced, dysmetria and adiadochokinesia are observed. Sometimes patients complain of sharp pain in the legs or lower back and involuntary muscle trembling. Muscle power in the extremities is significantly reduced, muscle tone is spastically increased, most often in the legs. Tendon reflexes are lively, pathologic reflexes are positive. Eye movement disorders are often discovered: ptosis, paresis of the abducens nerve, impaired convergence, sometimes optic atrophy, narrowing of the visual field, reduced visual acuity, positive Argyll-Robertson's sign. Extrapyramidal symptoms develop sometimes. Almost all patients have mental disturbances: intellectual decline and depressive disorders.

Diagnosis and differential diagnosis. Diagnosis is based on positive family history, cerebellar ataxia, increased tendon reflexes, eye movement disorders. EEG finds diffuse changes, consisting of delta- and theta-waves, with reduction of the alpha-rhythm. CT shows atrophy of the cerebellum and brain stem. Amino acid metabolism is affected: the concentration of leucine and alanine is decreased and their urinary excretion is reduced. Some rudiment forms of the disease, exhibiting symptoms characteristic of spinal atrophy or familial spastic paraplegia, present difficulties in differential diagnosis. The main distinction from Friedreich's Disease is the pattern of inheritance /dominant in cerebellar ataxia and recessive in Friedreich's Disease/ and the changes in tendon reflexes, which are weak or absent in Friedreich's Disease and increased in cerebellar ataxia. Moreover in cerebellar ataxia the onset is at a later age, skeletal deformities and sensory disturbances are infrequent, whereas they are characteristic of Friedreich's Disease. Dementia and eye movement disorders are more frequent with Pierre-Marie's disease. Multiple sclerosis, for which cerebellar, pyramidal and eye movement disturbances are characteristic, can also be hard to differentiate. It is distinguished by its remitting course, disturbances of sphincter control, temporal paleness of papillae, CSF changes, disappearance of superficial abdominal reflexes, etc.

Evolution. The course of the disease is constantly progressive. Various infections and intoxications, as well as other disorders, have a negative influence on the final outcome.

Treatment. It is symptomatic and general supportive: vitamins B1, B6, B12, nootropic medications /Nootropil, Aminalon, Cerebrolysin/, anticholinesterase agents /Proserine, Galantamine, Oxazyl/. Treatment with these drugs continues for approximately two months after which there are 3-4 month intervals of rest. Special rehabilitation is carried out, aimed at correction of coordination disturbances.

Prophylaxis. Genetic counseling.

2.2. Holmes' Olivo-cerebellar Atrophy.

Some authors identify this form with the "late Pierre-Marie's cerebellar atrophy". The dystrophic process affects mostly the cerebellar vermis and more slightly the cerebellar hemispheres. Degenerative changes also involve the olives. The pons and spinal cord are not affected. the disease begins around 40 years of age. The main clinical feature is ataxia originating in the vermis. Neocerebellar symptoms are added with involvement of the olives in the pathologic process /74/. The course of the disease is chronic progressive.

2.3. Olivo-ponto-cerebellar Atrophies.

Chronic progressive degenerative disorders characterized mainly by cerebellar disturbances. These diseases are heterogenous according to etiopathogenesis and include sporadic, as well as hereditary forms. Hereditary forms can be transmitted both in autosomal dominant and in autosomal recessive pattern /22, 82/.

Atrophy of cerebellar white matter is discovered pathomorpholigically, more pronounced in the hemispheres with intact nuclei. Degeneration of the olives, olivo-cerebellar tracts, ventral nuclei of pons and middle cerebellar peduncle is present. Degenerative processes later affect also the cerebellar cortex with involvement of Purkinje cells. Sometimes substantia nigra, tracts and posterior roots of the spinal cord, the frontal and temporal lobe of the brain, the nuclei of cranial nerves, etc. also become involved.

2.3.1.Dejerine-Thomas Olivo-ponto-cerebellar Atrophy.

A chronic, slowly progressing disorder, characterized mainly by cerebellar disturbances.

Synonyms. Dejerine-Thomas syndrome, atrophy of pons, presenile cerebellar atrophy, intracerebellar atrophy.

Etiology and pathogenesis. Not well clarified. The disorder sometimes develops in chronic alcohol abuse. Neurolues is assumed to have a role also. The disorder is heterogenous and there are both sporadic and hereditary forms. The latter can be transmitted both in autosomal dominant and in autosomal recessive pattern.

Pathomorphology. The dystrophic process is largely spread. The cerebellar cortex, inferior olive, nuclei and tracts in the brain stem and especially in the middle cerebellar peduncle, as well as the striopallidal system are affected. Dense glia expands in place of dead neurons.

Clinical manifestations. The major manifestations of the disorder are cerebellar disturbances. The sporadic form begins at the age of 35-40 years. First gait and upright position are affected. In the sitting and standing position marked oscillating body movements are observed. The gait becomes hesitating, broad-legged and patients often fall. In late stages of the disease they cannot move or turn around in bed. Ataxia in the extremities presents later and is slightly expressed. Movements become clumsy, dysmetria, adiadochokinesia, tremor and disturbed hand-writing are noted. Speech becomes slow, explosive, dysarthric. Horizontal nystagmus is often seen. Tendon and periostal reflexes are usually pathologically increased. Urine incontinence is registered. Mental and emotional disorders are frequent: lethargy, indifference, memory and intellectual fading. Agitation, disturbed consciousness, fears and hallucinations may appear. Extrapyramidal rigidity, dysarthria, amimia, hypobradykinesia, bulbar dysfunction develops in late stages of the disease.

Evolution. The prognosis is poor. The disease progresses to complete invalidization for 4-5 years and patients die or intercurrent infections.

Hereditary forms of olivo-ponto-cerebellar atrophy are divided into five major types:

Type I - Menzel type olivo-ponto-cerebellar degeneration. It is inherited in autososmal dominant pattern. The disease is manifested at the age of 11-60 years. The course is slow, progressive. The clinical manifestations include cerebellar symptoms /ataxia, muscle hypotonia, scanned speech with elements of dysarthria and intention tremor/, signs of damage to the caudal group of cranial nerves /dysarthria, dysphagia, dysphonia/. Subcortical ganglia are also affected /hyperkinesias/ and more rarely ocular motility nerves and posterior roots.

Type II – Fickler-Winkler type olivo-ponto-cerebellar degeneration. It is inherited in autosomal recessive pattern. It presents during the age of 20-80 years with symptoms of cerebellar damage, predominantly ataxia of the extremities. Sense perception and tendon reflexes are not normal. There are no pareses.

Type III - olivo-ponto-cerebellar degeneration with retinal degeneration. It is inherited in autososmal dominant pattern. It appears in youth. Along with cerebellar and extrapyramidal symptoms, there is progressive decline in visual acuity to complete blindness due to pigmentary retinopathy. Ophthalmoplegia and nystagmus are sometimes registered.

Type IV- Schut-Haymaker type olivo-ponto-cerebellar atrophy. It is inherited in autososmal dominant pattern. It begins in childhood. Along with cerebellar symptoms, there are signs of damage to the VII, IX, X and XII cranial nerves /facial nerve paralysis, bulbar symptoms/ and to the dorsal columns of the spinal cord /disturbed position and vibration sense/.

Type V - olivo-ponto-cerebellar degeneration with dementia, ophthalmoplegia and extrapyramidal symptoms. The pattern of inheritance is autosomal dominant.it develops in middle age. Along with cerebellar structures, substantia nigra, the nuclei of eye movement nerves and neurons of the frontal lobe of the cerebral hemispheres are also involved in the pathologic process. The form goes with dementia, progressive ophthalmoplegia, extrapyramidal symptoms /Parkinson-like syndrome/ and cerebellar disturbances.

Diagnosis and differential diagnosis. The diagnosis of olivo-ponto-cerebellar atrophy is confirmed by the characteristic clinical manifestations and CT: atrophy of the cerebellum and/or pons is seen, sometimes hydrocephalus. As a differential diagnosis one should consider: Friedreich's Disease, Pierre-Marie's disease, Refsum's disease, cerebellar tumors and early manifestations of Parkinsonism. The disease is differentiated from disseminated sclerosis by the continuous progression of symptoms, the absence of ocular motility problems in the sporadic form of olivo-ponto-cerebellar atrophy and the lack of changes in the CSF.

Evolution. The disorder progresses slowly but continuously. Patients die within a few years of intercurrent infections.

Treatment. Stimulators of brain metabolism are used: Pyramem, Aminalon, Cerebrolysin, vitamins B. rehabilitation is aimed at improving the coordination of movements. Anticholinesterase agents are used when extrapyramidal hyperkinesias develop.

2.4. R. Hunt's Dento-rubral Atrophy.

A chronic progressive disorder, characterized by cerebellar symptoms and predominantly intention tremor and myoclonic hyperkinesias, often with concurrent epileptic seizures.

Synonyms. Hunt's myoclonic cerebellar dyssinergia, Hunt's syndrome, dyssynergia cerebellaris progressive, atrophia dentorubralis, dyssynergia cerebellaris myoclonica.

Etiology and pathogenesis. The disorder is hereditary and is transmitted in autosomal recessive pattern, but sporadic cases are also described.

Pathomorphology. Degenerative changes in nucleus dentatus and nucleus ruber and superior cerebellar peduncles are characteristic of myoclonic cerebellar dyssynergia. Other cerebellar nuclei are also often involved in the pathologic process.

Clinical manifestations. The disease begins between 10 and 20 years of age with cerebellar symptomatics which is very intense during the whole course. Coarse intention tremor is characteristic and it is particularly expressed in the arms. Other cerebellar dysfunctions also appear often: ataxia, impaired coordination, speech problems, muscle hypotonia. Cerebellar disturbances gradually progress, myoclonic trembling and frequently epileptic seizures are added. The latter are not an obligatory feature of the disorder, and whenever they are present most often they are not of the grand mal type and rather exhibit the characteristics of complex partial seizures. Certain intellectual decline is noted. Sometimes a combination of manifestations of cerebellar myoclonic dyssynergia and symptoms characteristic of Friedreich's Disease is encountered.

A genetic variant of the disorder with dominant pattern of inheritance in 2-3 generations has been described. This form is different in its benign course, absence of mental alterations and infrequency of epileptic seizures.

Diagnosis and differential diagnosis. Hunt's disease must be distinguished from myoclonus epilepsy of the Unverricht-Lundborg type in which cerebellar symptoms might be observed. They, however, are weak. The cardinal features of myoclonus epilepsy are the wide-spread myoclonic hyperkinesias and epileptic seizures. In cerebellar dyssynergia extrapyramidal rigidity does not develop in contrast to myoclonus epilepsy, and personality degradation is not always present. In Hunt's disease the course is progressive and not remitting, there are no pyramidal and eye movement disorders, impaired sphincter control or pathology in CSF in contrast to multiple sclerosis.

Cerebellar dyssynergia is differentiated from Friedreich's ataxia by the absence of sensory disturbances, areflexia, nystagmus and intense intention tremor.

Evolution. The disorder progresses slowly and continuously. Patients die of intercurrent infections within a few years.

Treatment. It is symptomatic. Phenobarbital, benzodiazepines, vitamins, nootropic medications, etc. are used.

Prophylaxis. Genetic counseling.

2.5. Marinescu-Sjogren Syndrome.

A chronic progressive disorder which is characterized clinically by the triad cerebellar ataxia-mental retardation-cataract.

Synonyms. Congenital cataract, mental retardation and ataxia. Marinescu-Sjogren-Garland syndrome.

Etiology and pathogenesis. It is inherited in autosomal recessive pattern. There is a high percentage /approximately 60%/ of consanguinity.

Pathomorphology. There is atrophy of the cerebellum, degeneration of the inferior olives, the pons nuclei and lesser of the pyramidal tracts.

Clinical manifestations. There is a classical triad of symptoms: cerebellar dysfunction /ataxia, dysmetria and intention tremor/, congenital cataract and mental retardation together with retardation in physical development. These clinical manifestations develop in different sequence: sometimes mental retardation is the debut, in other cases the cataract or coordination disturbances. In some instances other pathological changes are found: bone abnormalities /kyphoscoliosis, high-arched feet, dolichocephaly/, trophic disturbances, deafness, sexual dysfunction, epileptic seizures, gaze paralyses, strabismus, nystagmus, etc. at autopsy of patients encephalopathy and renal tubule necrosis are discovered.

Treatment. Symptomatic.

2.6. Bassen-Kornzweig Syndrome. /Abetalipoproteinemia/.

A chronic progressive degenerative disorder characterized by cerebellar ataxia, pigmentary retinopathy, mental retardation and steatorrhoea.

Synonyms. Ataxia progressive, pigmentary retinopathy, acantocytosis.

Etiology and pathogenesis. Autosomal recessive disease which develops in the age of 2 to 16 years. The pathogenesis is related to vitamin E deficiency and low cholesterol level.

Pathomorphology. The morphological substrate of the syndrome is demyelinization of spinocerebellar tracts, dorsal columns and cerebellar peduncles. Cardiomegaly and manifestations of heart failure are registered. Erythrocytes show deformities: acanthocytosis /they have "thorny" cell surface with projecting spicules/ /43/.

Clinical manifestations. It resembles the clinical manifestations of Friedreich's Disease. The features of cerebellar ataxia /ataxia of the extremities and body, dysarthria and nystagmus/ are specific. Often mental development is impaired but this is not obligatory. Signs of polyneuropathy with atrophy of peroneal muscles are observed.

Paraclinical investigations demonstrate steatorrhoea, decreased level of cholesterol, carotins, vitamin A and phospholipids. There are no β-lipoproteins.

Treatment. The diet is low-fat because of the steatorrhoea, and administration of vitamin E slows the progression of the disease and the manifestations of polyneuropathy.

2.7. Louis-Bar Syndrome.

A hereditary disorder from the group of phakomatoses which is characterized by cerebellar ataxia, teleangiectasia and susceptibility to recurrent infections.

Synonyms. Ataxia teleangiectatica, Boder-Sedwik syndrome, oculocutaneous cerebellar teleangiectasia, atrophy of the cerebellum with oculocutaneous teleangiectasias and bronchiectases, ataxia teleangiectasia syndrome.

Etiology and pathogenesis. The disorder is hereditary and is transmitted in autosomal recessive pattern. The mutant gene has high penetrance. Louis-Bar Syndrome is a immunodeficiency disorder. Hypoplasia of the thymus and hypogammaglobulinemia often occur and mostly the level of immunoglobulin E and/or A is decreased. In some cases a chromosomal abnormality is established: translocation between two acrocentric chromosomes of groups 13-14-15. Poor vascularization of the skin, conjunctivae and brain is inherited /85/.

Pathomorphology. Primary degeneration of the cerebellar cortex, predominantly Purkinje cells and the granular layer with subsequent atrophy of the white matter.

Clinical manifestations. The disorder begins in early childhood with atactic disturbances which slowly progress and patients become completely handicapped around 10 years of age. Certain improvement of motor functions is described at the age of 2-5 years which is explained with compensatory effect of growing motor abilities. In a number of cases besides atactic manifestations, extrapyramidal disturbances are also observed: hypokinesias, athetosic or myoclonic hyperkinesias, damage to the cranial nerves, weak tendon reflexes and mental retardation. Teleangiectasias present at approximately 3 years of age, first on the bulbi: in the bulbar conjunctivae, afterwards they may spread on the skin of the face, trunk and extremities. There is a tendency for recurrences of infectious diseases mainly of the upper respiratory tract and lungs: sinusitis, rhinitis, tonsillitis and bronchopneumonia which are related to immune deficiency. In patients with Louis-Bar Syndrome there is dysfunction of cellular and humoral immunity simultaneously as a result of hypoplasia of the thyroid gland. Deficiency of T-dependent lymphocytes and immunoglobulins A and E is characteristic of the disease. The high risk of malignant disorders in ataxia teleangiectasia is associated with this.

Diagnosis and differential diagnosis. The diagnosis is made on the basis of the characteristic combination of cerebellar atactic manifestations and teleangiectasias. CT shows cerebellar atrophies. Differential diagnosis is made with the other variants of cerebellar atrophy. Furthermore one should have in mind Sturge-Weber disease /in it there is nevus flammeus on the face and head, epileptic seizures and congenital glaucoma/, Hippel-Lindau disease /it goes with angiomatosis of the retina, cerebellum and internal organs; cerebellar manifestations are homolateral to the localization of the angiomatosis; vision is severely impaired/; Bonnet-Dechaume-Blanc disease /it manifests with retinal and mesencephalic angiomatosis, homonymous hemianopsia, exophthalmus and decreased visual acuity, and pyramidal signs are found on the contralateral side/, etc.

Evolution. The disorder is slowly progressive. It is often complicated by intercurrent infections.

Treatment. General supportive and symptomatic agents.

Prophylaxis. Genetic counseling. Secondary prophylaxis of infectious and malignant diseases.

2.8. Refsum Disease.

A hereditary degenerative disorder with various clinical course, the most characteristic manifestations of which are cerebellar ataxia, chronic distal polyneuropathy and pigmentary retinopathy.

Synonyms. Heredoataxia polyneuritiformis, heredopathia atactica polyneuritiformis, heredopathia hemeralopica polyneuritiformis.

Frequency. The disorder is rare; there are 100 cases described for certain. The initial gene mutation is supposed to have originated in the Scandinavian countries and from there to have spread elsewhere. The disorder affects all ages, but it is encountered most frequently between 10 and 30 years of age.

Etiology and pathogenesis. The disease is inherited in autosomal recessive pattern but there are also sporadic cases. The pathogenesis is associated with blockage of normal oxidation of phytanic acid into α-hydroxy-phytanic acid which leads to accumulation of phytanic acid in blood and tissues. The primary defect is the congenital deficiency of α-hydroxylase of phytanic acid: an enzyme localized in mitochondria. Under normal conditions phytanic acid, which is one of the fatty acids, is not synthesized in the body and is provided from fat-containing foods.

Pathomorphology. Severe fat degeneration of peripheral nerves and less pronounced degeneration in the medulla oblongata, pons and cerebellum. Pia mater is fibrous dense.

Clinical manifestations. The course of the disease is slow. The major clinical manifestation is chronic distal sensory-motor polyneuropathy. Other characteristic symptoms are cerebellar ataxia and atypical pigment degeneration of the retina which goes as pigmentary retinopathy. Night blindness and limited visual field is often seen. Other concurrent disorders are cataract, anosmia, deafness, skeletal deformity, and ichthyosis on the feet, palms and body. Epiphyseal dysplasia is also found. The development of cardiomyopathy may lead to sudden death of patients /71/.

Diagnosis and differential diagnosis. The diagnosis is made on the basis of the most typical clinical manifestations. Paraclinical investigations are of great importance. Very high level of the fatty phytanic acid is found in serum. EMG usually shows decreased conduction velocity on nerve branches. In CSF there is protein cell dissociation with elevation of β- and γ-globulins. ECG changes include sinus tachycardia, inversion of the waves, disturbed conduction. Differential diagnosis is made most often with Guillain-Barre polyneuritis /it has the characteristics of an infectious disease/, with Dejerine-Sotas polyneuritis /in it there are no cerebellar manifestations or pigment degeneration of the retina/ and neural muscular atrophy /there are no cerebellar symptoms, patient's legs look like "bottles turned upside down"/. In all the three diseases there is n phytanic acid in the serum.

Evolution. The course of the disease is slow with remissions.

Treatment. Strict adherence to the diet is very important: avoidance of foods containing dairy products or meat.

Prophylaxis. Genetic counseling. Because of the low incidence of the disorder, in suspicious cases it is necessary to check the level of phytanic acid in serum.

Chapter IV

NEUROLIPIDOSES AND LEUKODYSTROPHIES

Neurolipidoses and leukodystrophies are hereditary /most often autosomal recessive/ disorders of the nervous system which go like dysmetabolic encephalopathies and appear mainly in childhood.

Their course is quite similar; often there are forms that are hard to differentiate, because of which a series of biochemical and morphological tests are required besides clinical observation. In this sense the differentiation between lipidoses and leukodystrophies is rather arbitrary /1, 3, 7, 9/.

Neurolipidoses. Neurolipidoses are hereditary disorders caused by accumulation of lipids in the cells of the nervous system leading to their death. A number of diseases are included in this group, which as a rule present in childhood. In most of them there is a defective mechanism of ferment metabolism of fats.

1. Gangliosidoses.

Gangliosidoses belong to the group of sphingolipidoses.

Sphingolipids are the major lipid brain constituent which includes gangliosides /complexes of lipids with sialic acid/, cerebrosides, sulfatides and sphingomyelin. Biochemically, according to the deposited substance in the brain tissue, we distinguish:

a/ Gm_2-gangliosidosis /G - ganglioside, m - monosialoside, the subindex 2 – type ceramide/, known as Tay-Sachs;

b/ Gm_1-gangliosidosis, known as Norman-Landing and Derry's disease;

c/ Gm_3-gangliosidosis;

1.1. Tay-Sachs Disease /Gm2-Gangliosidosis, Variant B/.

A hereditary degenerative disorder which is characterized by delayed psychomotor development, bilateral retinal atrophy and macrocephaly.

Synonyms. Gangliocellular heredodegenerative idiocy, familial amaurotic idiocy, Tay-Knigdon syndrome.

Etiology and pathogenesis. Deficiency of hexosaminidase A in tissues and body fluids and increased activity of hexosaminidase B is transmitted in autosomal recessive pattern. The disorder is more frequent in Jewish children. Fructose 1-phosphate aldolase is decreased in serum in both patients and their parents. Increased activity of some enzymes is found in CSF: mainly hydrogenases.

Pathomorphology. Morphological examination demonstrates macro- and sometimes microcephaly. Gross changes in the brain are not seen. Sometimes it is a bit enlarged or reduced in size; the cerebellum shows slight atrophy. To the contrary, there are characteristic changes in the cells of the cerebral cortex. The cytoplasm is enlarged, filled with sudanophilic Sudan III, Sudanschwartz and PAS-positive substance. At enzymatic investigation for acid phosphatase, a positive reaction is read. Under the electron microscope the inclusions in the cellular cytoplasm look like concentric laminar bodies: membranous cytoplasmic bodies. They are found in the neurons of the central nervous system and in the ganglial cells of the autonomic nervous system and some internal organs. The substance accumulated in the cells is Gm2-gasnglioside.

Clinical manifestations. The disorder begins at approximately 3-6 months of age following a normal pregnancy and delivery. First a delay in motor and cognitive milestones is observed, which quickly grows into profound mental retardation. In the beginning muscles are hypotonic, but eventually severe rigidity develops. At the age of 3-4 months hyperacusis appears, which is provoked by the slightest noises. Towards the end of the first year in 95% of cases ophthalmoscopic examination finds a red spot in the retina due to the atrophy; visual acuity declines to complete amaurosis. Acquired motor skills are lost rapidly; microcephaly progresses. In the terminal stages of the disorder the children are blind, with quadriparesis, dementia, epileptic seizures and severe autonomic disturbances develop. Death of intercurrent diseases occurs within 2 years from the initiation of the symptoms.

1.2. Sandhoff Disease /Gm2-Gangliosidosis, Variant 0/.

The simultaneous lack of both hexosaminidase A and B is characteristic of this disorder. It occurs in non-Jewish races. The disease is morphologically similar to Tay-Sachs Disease except for the presence of foamy histiocytes in some organs, including the bone marrow. The substance accumulated is Gm2-gasnglioside. The disorder begins at approximately 1-2 years of age and its course does not differ substantially from Tay-Sachs Disease. It progresses a little bit slower /5-9 years/ and with mild hepatosplenomegaly.

1.3. Bernheimer-Seitelberg Disease /Gm2-Gangliosidosis, Juvenile Variant 0/.

It begins a little bit later, between 4 and 6 years of age. Atrophy of the brain and internal organs is found morphologically. There is no red spot in the retina, nor hepatosplenomegaly. In the cells of the CNS there are cytoplasmic inclusions similar to the ones in Tay-Sachs Disease, but lipofuscin granules are also found, associated with dense aggregates. The major clinical manifestation is locomotor ataxia; spasticity to decerebration rigidity develops, as well as loss of the ability to speak. This disorder progresses more slowly, for 5-15 years.

4.4. Gm2-Gangliosidosis, Variant AB.

This disorder does not differ from Tay-Sachs Disease in anything else but the normal amount of hexosaminidase A and B.

4.5. Generalized Monosialogangliosidosis Gm1 / Gangliosidosis Gm1, Normann-Landig Type I/.

It develops as a result of excessive accumulation of gangliosides and mucopolysaccharides in neurons, internal organs and bones. Inclusions are found in hepatocytes, Kupfer cells, renal glomeruli, peripheral nerves and vascular endothelium, and foamy cells are discovered in bone marrow. Electron microscopic changes are the same as in Tay-Sachs Disease. A coarse grotesque face, macroglossia, hepatosplenomegaly, flexion contractures of joints, muscle hypotonia, tonic-clonic seizures, severe mental retardation are observed clinically. The course is rapid and progressive, for 2-3 years.

4.6.   Generalized Gm1- Gangliosidosis Type II /Derey/.
The pathomorphologic changes are the same as the ones in the first form. The disorder manifests clinically during the 2nd year of life with ataxia and hypotonia, which later turns into severe muscle rigidity, with epileptic seizures, decerebration and death after 7-8 years.

4.7.   Gm3-Gangliosidosis.
A very rare disorder. Biochemically it is characterized by a defect in the biosynthesis and to a lesser degree in the metabolism of gangliosides. Its clinical manifestations include macroglossia, high arched palate, epileptic seizures, dementia and slow evolution.

Diagnosis and differential diagnosis. Antenatal diagnosis of Tay-Sachs Disease is possible by measuring the activity of hexosaminidase A in amniotic fluid, which shows a low level. As a differential diagnosis Laurence-Moon-Biedl syndrome is most important to be recognized; obesity, polydactyly and sexual infantilism are characteristic of it. Forms with later onset must be distinguished from cerebellar and hereditary extrapyramidal disorders / Friedreich's Disease, myoclonus epilepsy, etc./. In such cases the coexistence of cerebellar or extrapyramidal syndromes with mental retardation and alterations in the fundi of the eyes is of great importance for the diagnosis.

Evolution. These disorders progress for a few years and end with death of intercurrent diseases.

Treatment. Symptomatic. Vitamins, nootropic medications, enzyme preparations, plasma, etc. are used, with no substantial effect.

Prophylaxis. Genetic counseling. In case of decreased level of hexosaminidase A in amniotic fluid, pregnancy interruption is advised.

2. Cerebrosidoses.

A group of disorders associated with disturbed metabolism of cerebrosides is known under this name. Cerebrosides is the generic name of a group of ceramide monohexosides /glucocerebrosides and galactocerebroside/. Gaucher Disease and Fabry Disease fall into this category.

2.1. Gaucher Disease.

A hereditary degenerative disorder characterized by hepatosplenomegaly, muscle rigidity and progressive dementia.

Synonyms. Cerebrosidosis, keratin type lipid histiocytosis, Gaucher type giant cell splenomegaly, primary idiopathic splenomegaly, Gaucher-Schlegenhaufer syndrome, glucocerebrosidosis.

Etiology and pathogenesis. Deficiency of glucocerebrosidase – an enzyme, breaking down glucocerebroside into glucose and ceramide – inherited in autosomal recessive pattern.
Lipid metabolism is disturbed leading to accumulation of cerebrosides in the cells of the nervous system and some internal organs.

Pathomorphology. Neuronal death is found in the brain. There is accumulation of glucocerebroside in the reticuloendothelial system, perivascularly, in the bone marrow. Gaucher cells are typical for the disorder: large macrophages with eccentric one or several small nuclei. The cytoplasm is PAS-positive, MB-negative and slightly sudanophilic. The reaction for acid phosphatase is positive. Such cells are found around brain vessels, in lymph nodes and the bone marrow. Groups of tubular profiles 200-300 micrones in diameter are found under the electron microscope.

Clinical manifestations. There are 3 clinical variants: acute infantile malignant form, juvenile form and chronic form in adults.

The infantile form begins early and leads to death within 2 years. As a result of deposition of lipids in the spleen, liver and brain, hepatosplenomegaly, delay in cognitive development, epileptic seizures, spastic pareses and paralyses develop.

In the juvenile form there is severe dementia and various hyperkinesias along with seizures and spastic pareses.

The chronic form in adults is characterized by scanty neurologic symptomatics and more pronounced manifestations from the internal organs: a large belly, splenomegaly, yellow-brown spots on the skin, infantilism, hemorrhagic diatheses, aseptic bone necroses, bronchopneumonias, which can become complicated with cor pulmonale. Pyramidal symptoms and epileptic seizures are rare. In such cases the CBC shows hypochromic anemia, thrombocytopenia, leucopenia and expansion of Gaucher cells in the bone marrow.

The diagnosis is made by establishment of deficiency of the enzyme glucocerebrosidase and by biopsy of the sural nerve, the colon or the brain. Sometimes CSF demonstrates moderately increased protein level. Differential diagnosis: most often with Niemann-Pick Disease.

Treatment. Symptomatic.

2.2. Fabry Disease.

A very rare degenerative disorder characterized by joint pain, angiectasias and pyramidal signs.

Synonyms. Fabry glycosphingolipidosis, angiokeratoma corporis diffusa.

Etiology and pathogenesis. The disorder is inherited in X-linked recessive type and is due to α-galactoside hydrolase deficiency /19/.

Pathomorphology. There is vacuolization of the muscular layer in vessel walls and hypertrophy of myocardial fibers. Lipid deposition is found in ganglial cells of the brain and peripheral nerves, in renal tubules and in lymph nodes. Osmiphilic membranous and lamellar deposits are seen under the electron microscope.

Clinical manifestations. Paroxysmal joint pain, sometimes abdominal pain or backache, together with fever and increased ESR often occur in childhood. Autonomic disturbances are also typical. The pain is related to the involvement of the spinal ganglia and nerve branches. Skin changes are characteristic for the disease: angiokeratoma and teleangiectasias. They affect the lower part of the body as red-violet nodules. The cornea becomes turbid. Nephropathy and cardiopathy develop, which shows the characteristics of angina pectoris or myocardial infarction. Brain insults may also occur around the 20th year of age. Neurologic examination demonstrates nistagmus, pareses, paresthesias, often headache. Cognitive development is sometimes delayed.

Diagnosis and differential diagnosis. The diagnosis is made after finding the characteristic crystalloid lipid inclusions in a biopsy specimen from internal organs. Several forms of disseminated sclerosis must be considered as the most important differential diagnosis.

Evolution. The course of the disease is slow, progressive. Patients can live up to 40 years of age, when they die of recurring infections, renal failure combined with anemia or myocardial infarction.

Treatment. Symptomatic.

Prophylaxis. Genetic counseling. In those at risk, interruption of pregnancy is recommended.

3. Sphingomyelinoses.

Disorders associated with involvement of sphingomyelin. It is a primary group of sphingosine, esterified with choline phosphate.

3.1. Niemann-Pick Disease.

A degenerative disorder from the group of lipidoses, characterized by hepatosplenomegaly, cachexia, progressive mental retardation, motor disturbances and frequently blindness.

Synonyms. Lipoid cell hepatosplenomegaly, reticular and histiocyte sphingomyelinosis; essential lipoid histiocytosis, phosphatide lipoidosis.

Etiology and pathogenesis. A defect in the metabolism of sphingomyelin is inherited in autosomal recessive pattern, leading to its accumulation in the tissues of the reticuloendothelial system and the brain. Deficiency of the enzyme sphingomyelinase, which catalyzes the separation of phosphorylcholine from ceramide, plays a primary role in the pathogenesis. When there is deficiency of sphingomyelinase A, the brain is affected, and when there is deficiency of sphingomyelinase B, it is not injured.

Pathomorphology. Hepatosplenomegaly is characteristic. Lymph nodes are enlarged. The brain is reduced in size, the gyri are atrophic and the sulci are wider. Microscopic examination reveals "Niemann-Pick" cells: they have a centrally or peripherally located nucleus and cytoplasm filled with granular substance. Some call them "foamy cells" and they can be seen in all organs. The presence of sphingomyelin can be established in them. Under the electron microscope neurons contain bright vacuoles, surrounded by a simple membrane and there are concentric membranes in their center.

Clinical manifestations. There are 4 forms of the disease:

- Type A. Infantile form. The reason for it is a defect of sphingomyelinase A. It begins in the first year of life with a delay in motor and cognitive milestones, progressive dementia, hepatosplenomegaly, a red spot in the macula is found in half of the children. Patients die before the 3rd year mainly of interstitial pneumonias.
- Type B. Chronic form. The reason for it is a deficiency of sphingomyelinase B. It is characterized by hepatosplenomegaly without brain damage.
- Type C. Subacute form. In this case there is no a deficiency of sphingomyelinase. It begins in adolescence or adulthood and is distinguished by a benign course, later occurrence of neurologic symptoms and insignificant enlargement of the liver and spleen.
- Type D. New Scottish form. It follows an atypical course with a later onset, slow evolution and manifestations mainly from the liver: subacute hepatitis and cirrhosis; the nervous system is not affected.

Diagnosis and differential diagnosis. The establishment of Niemann-Pick cells in biopsy specimen from internal organs is important for making the diagnosis along with the clinical course. In the aspect of differential diagnosis the disorder must be distinguished from other lipidoses and internal diseases with hepatosplenomegaly: hepatitis, cirrhosis, malignant blood disorders, some parasitic diseases, etc.

Evolution. Dependingt on the clinical form the disease continues from 3 years to middle or older age.

Treatment. Symptomatic.

Prophylaxis. Genetic counseling.

4. Mucopolysaccharidoses and Mucolipidoses.

A joint group of diseases characterized by disturbed pathways of enzymes participating in the metabolism of glycosaminoglycans. Accumulation of glycosaminoglycans in cells and tissues and their excretion in urine result from these disturbances. The missing enzymes in the two subgroups are different. Moreover in mucopolysaccharidoses there is excretion of mucopolysaccharides in urine whereas there is no such excretion in mucolipidoses. The clinical characteristics of the two subgroups, however, are quite similar, because of which they are discussed together.

4.1. Mucopolysaccharidoses.

A group of disorders associated with genetic disturbances in the breakage of acid mucopolysaccharides, caused by specific enzyme deficiency. They affect connective tissue and manifest with damages to the locomotory system, internal organs, vision and nervous system /84/.

4.1.1. Hurler's Disease /Mucopolysaccharidosis Type I/.

A hereditary disorder from the group of mucopolysaccharidoses which is characterized by a grotesque figure, hepatosplenomegaly, visual disturbances and intellectual deficit.

Synonyms. Gargoylism, Lipochondrodystrophia, disostosis multiplex, Thompson syndrome, multiple dysostosis, dysostotic idiocy, familial dysostosic "dwarfism", mucopolysaccharidosis.

Etiology and pathogenesis. It is inherited in an autosomal recessive pattern. Deficiency of the ferment α-L-iduronidase lies in basis of the pathogenesis and leads to disturbance of the catabolism of dermatansulfate and heparansulfate. These mucopolysaccharides accumulate in cells and are excreted in urine.

Pathomorphology. At pathomorphologic examination mucopolysaccharide accumulation in the form of granular substance in the parenchyma of the liver, spleen, renal tubules, retina, sclera and cornea is seen. Deposits of that kind are also found in nervous cells, the intima of the coronary arteries, the bronchi, etc. Brain tissue shows atrophies, more intense for the white matter, in which there is gliosis. Neurons have a ballooned cytoplasm, the nucleus is pushed to the periphery. Multivesicular inclusions are discovered under the electron microscope. Internal hydrocephalus may develop; sometimes the cerebellum is also affected.

Clinical manifestations. Characteristic of the disease are a grotesque figure with a big head, coarse facial features, thick and inversely turned lips, macroglossia, thick eyebrows and wide nares. The neck is short, the body is stumpy, with comparatively long extremities, broad hands resembling paws; limited mobility of large joints; thickened skin. Breathing becomes difficult due to hyperplasia of nasal mucosa; there is hepatosplenomegaly, turbid cornea, often deafness. Cardiopathies develop because of thickening of the heart valves. Cognitive development is delayed, epileptic seizures are observed. Patients are noisy, sometimes aggressive.

Diagnosis and differential diagnosis. The diagnosis is made by testing the urine with toluidine blue, staining the material with toluidine blue also, quantitative determination of mucopolysaccharides via electrophoresis following extraction, evaluation of the enzymes in tissue cultures, examination of the skin under electron microscope. Roentgenographic examination shows elongated and oblique sella turcica, curved long bones, lumbar vertebra look like spurs and are deformed. Differential diagnosis is made with other diseases of this group and with mucolipidoses.

Evolution. The course of the disorder is malignant. Patients die within less than 10 years.

Treatment. Plasma transfusion is applied, as well as fibroblast transplantation, but with no substantial effect.

Prophylaxis. Genetic counseling. Antenatal diagnosis is made by examining the concentration and distribution of acid mucopolysaccharides in amniotic fluid and by adding radioactive sulfate to amniotic cell cultures.

4.1.2. Hunter's Syndrome /Mucopolysaccharidosis Type II/.

The recessive pathologic gene is localized in the X-chromosome as a result of which predominantly males suffer from the disease. In rare instances the disorder may develop in girls as well, probably as a homozygous presentation occurring as a result of a de novo mutation in the X-chromosome received from the father.

The syndrome is caused by deficiency of the enzyme L-indurono-sulfate sulfatase, which breaks the nonorganic sulfate from induronic acid. Accumulation of dermatansulfate and heparansulfate occur here also, like in gargoylism, but in lesser amount.

Clinical symptoms develop after birth but are also less intense hen compared to the ones in Hurler's Disease. Deformities of the bones and skull are lighter. The cornea does not become turbid. Hepatosplenomegaly and cardiovascular disorders are moderately pronounced. There is, however, severe mental retardation. Skin changes are pathognomonic for this form: large areas of the skin are smooth, shining and with no hair on the background of general hirsutism and thickening of the skin.

The evolution is slow, progressive. Patients reach up to 30 years of age.

4.1.3. Sanfilippo Syndrome /Mucopolysaccharidosis Type III/.

This is a heterogenous group of clinically similar forms, inherited in an autosomal recessive pattern, in which the metabolism of heparansulfate is disturbed.

Etiology and pathogenesis. Three subtypes are distinguished pathogenically: type IIIa, caused by deficiency of the enzyme heparin-N-sulfatase, type IIIb, cased by deficiency of the enzyme α-N-acetylglucosaminidase and type IIIc, caused by deficiency of the enzyme α-glucosaminidase.

Pathomorphology. Moderate hepatosplenomegaly, cerebral atrophy involving predominantly the white matter, slight atrophy of the cerebral cortex and dilated ventricles. Deposition of lipids in neurons and metachromatic substance in macrophages is detected histochemically.

Clinical manifestations. The disease presents during the 2nd-3rd year of life. Severe mental retardation and comparatively mild somatic problems is characteristic. Children are agitated, with attention deficit, sometimes aggressive. Speech develops difficultly; in some cases there is deafness. The grotesque face and hepatosplenomegaly are less marked.

Evolution. It follows a slow, progressive course. Patients reach 20-25 years of age.

4.1.4. Morquio Syndrome /Mucopolysaccharidosis Type IV/.

It is inherited in autosomal recessive pattern. The deficiency of the enzyme N-acetylhexosamine-6-SO4-sulfatase plays a crucial role in the pathogenesis of the diseases, leading to impaired hydrolysis of keratansulfate and to a lesser degree of dermatansulfate as well.

The disorder begins 1-2 years after birth. It is characterized by skeletal deformities, particularly of the spine and knees. The neck and trunk are short, the mandible is wide. Around the 10th year the cornea becomes turbid; aortic insufficiency and neurologic symptoms to quadriplegia are noted later, resulting from spinal cord compression from the spinal deformities. Intellect decline is mild and there are no skin changes.

4.1.5. Scheie Syndrome /Mucopolysaccharidosis Type V/.

It is inherited in autosomal recessive pattern. The syndrome is a result of a mutation in the gene which is heteroallelic to the gene responsible for Hurler's syndrome. The deficiency of the enzyme α-L-hyaluronidase lies in the basis of the disease.

Damages to the large and small joints of the lower extremities are leading among the clinical manifestations resulting in their deformation. Children are with an unusually big mouth and thickened skin, but intellect is not affected.

4.1.6. Maroteaux-Lamy Syndrome / Mucopolysaccharidosis Type VI/.

It is inherited in recessive pattern. The deficiency of the enzyme arylphosphatase B lies in the basis of the disease.

It begins during infancy. The leading symptoms are skeletal abnormalities and microcephaly. Joints have limited mobility. Hydrocephalus may develop. Predominantly heparansulfate is excreted in urine. Patients die mainly of pulmonary infections and heart failure for approximately 10-15 years.

4.1.7. H. Sly Syndrome

It is inherited in autosomal recessive pattern. In this case the metabolism of the three fractions of glycosaminoglycans is impaired because of deficiency of the ferment β-D-glucoronidase.

The characteristic grotesque face of the children is formed since birth. Intellect is reserved or moderately declined. They have a short stature; the liver and spleen enlarge in size. Pulmonary infections are frequent. The evolution is slow, progressive.

4.2. Mucolipidoses.

A heterogenic group of diseases the basis of which are lysosomal enzymatic defects, leading to accumulation of oligosaccharides and phospholipids in visceral, mesenchymal and nerve cells.

4.2.1. Mucolipidosis Type I /Sialidosis/.

It is inherited in autosomal recessive pattern. The disease is due to deficiency of the enzyme α-neuraminidase.

There is progressive dysmorphia like in Hurler's Syndrome but the excretion of mucopolysaccharides in urine is normal.

The initial clinical features appear during the second half of the first year of life with apparent delay in motor and cognitive development. There is kyphosis, muscle hypotonia, which subsequently turns into hypertonia, locomotor ataxia, myoclonus and seizures. A red spot might be seen in the macula. Hepatosplemegaly is not obligatory. Symptoms reminding of gargoylism are not always observed.

Metachromatic granules are found in cerebellar cells and peripheral lymphocytes, and bright vacuoles in hepatocytes. Urine testing detects oligosaccharides containing sialic acid. Roentgenologic examination shows skeletal disturbances similar to those in Sanfilippo Syndrome.

4.2.2. Mucolipidosis Type II /I-Cell-Disease/.

It is inherited in autosomal recessive pattern. There is deficiency of several lysosomal enzymes /hydrolases/ with accumulation of dermatansulfate in fibroblasts. Dark spherical inclusions are seen around the nuclei because of which the disease is also called I-Cell-Disease. No mucopolysaccharides are detected in urine.

He clinical course resembles Hurler's Syndrome, but the onset is from infancy and is more malignant. Patients are of short stature, dementia develops, joints become hard to move. Hepatomegaly and turbid cornea are rare. Respiratory infections are frequent. Roentgenographic examination of bones discovers changes analogous to those in Hurler's Syndrome.

Lethal outcome occurs within a few years of cardiovascular complications and pulmonary infections.

4.2.3. Mucolipidosis Type III /Pseudolipodystrophy/.

It is inherited in autosomal recessive pattern. The enzymatic defect is analogous to the one in type II but here it is less expressed.

Clinically defects of joints and muscles appear first /short stature, limited joint mobility, short neck, femoral dysplasia/. In approximately 6-7 years from birth a grotesque face may be observed but this is not obligatory. Progressive intellectual degradation develops gradually. Turbid cornea is also seen. Cardiac abnormalities, that decompensate around the 20th week, are not infrequent.

Roentgenologic examination demonstrates significant skeletal deformities, predominantly of the femurs, pelvis and spinal vertebra. These changes are more serious in boys in comparison to girls. Cells with vacuolized cytoplasm, containing glycolipids and acid Mucopolysaccharides are found in the bone marrow. A reduction in the activity of lysosomal hydrolases intracellularly, and an increase in their activity in plasma and in cultures of patient's cultivated cells are characteristic.

4.2.4. Mucolipidosis Type IV.

The inheritance of this form is autosomal recessive. The pathogenesis is not well understood.

The first clinical signs develop during the second half of the first year of life. In the beginning turbid corneas of both eyes and decreased vision are detected. Motor disturbances and a delay in psychomotor development are registered later.

Bone marrow biopsy demonstrates a large number of vacuolized histiocyte-like cells with lipid inclusions which show a slightly positive reaction for acid glycosaminoglycans.

The evolution is slow, progressive.

4.2.5. Fucosidosis.

This form is also inherited in autosomal recessive pattern. There is a defect in the metabolism of the enzyme α-L-fucosidase which takes part in the breakage of glycolipids. As a result, fucose-containing ceramide-oligohexosides accumulate in the liver and brain.

According to the clinical course there are two forms of the disease: infantile and juvenile.

The infantile form begins during infancy with muscle hypotonia, and spastic quadriparesis develops later. Motor and cognitive development is delayed and features of gargoylism may appear with diffuse angiokeratomas on the body. Tremor and slowed reactions to changes in the surroundings are noted. There is hepatosplenomegaly and susceptibility to recurrent infections. The duration of patients' life reaches up to 10 years.

The juvenile form begins during the 2nd year of life and develops more slowly. Here angiectaias, as well as all characteristic signs of mucopolysaccharidoses, are also typical. The quantity of sodium and chlorides in sweat is normal in contrast to the infantile form where it is increased. Patients live longer and can reach adulthood.

Roentgenologic examination demonstrates multiple mild dysostoses together with microcephaly, decreased transparence of cranial bones and hypoplasia of vertebral bodies.

Lymphocytes in peripheral blood are vacuolized. Inclusions containing sudanophil substances: glycolipids, are found in hepatocytes, Kupfer cells and some neurons.

4.2.6. Manosidosis.

It is inherited in autosomal recessive pattern. The almost complete absence of the enzyme α-manosidase in patients' brain, liver and spleen lies in the basis of the pathogenesis.

Pathomorphologic examination shows damage to the neurons of the cerebral cortex, brain stem and spinal cord. Increased concentration of acid mucopolysaccharides is found in them. Degenerative changes of myelin are detected in white matter.

Clinical manifestations. The first manifestations of the syndrome appear soon after birth: hepatosplenomegaly, muscle hypertonia and hyperreflexia. Infections of the upper airways are frequent. Signs of gargoylism may be observed during the 2nd year of life.

Widened ribs, coarse trabecularization of bones, oval vertebral bodies are found roentgenologically.

Lymphocytes in peripheral blood are vacuolized, the excretion of mucopolysaccharides in urine is normal or slightly increased.

The evolution is slow, progressive.

4.2.7. Rare forms.

Aspatrylglucosaminuria is a very rare disease with occurrence of dysmorphic features during school-age years, diarrhea, cataract and impaired hearing. Mucosulfatidosis. The latter develops when there is deficiency of sulfatases. Deficiency of the three isoferments of arylsulfatase A, which participates in the metabolism of sulfatized acid mucopolysaccharides and sphingolipids, lies in the basis of the pathogenesis of the disease. It is characterized clinically by delayed psychomotor development, facial grotesqueness which is not marked and spastic quadriparesis concomitant with tremor and myoclonus. There is no enlargement of the liver or spleen. Patients die before the onset of puberty.

5. Other Neurolipidoses.

A large group of various diseases , some of which are characterized by brain damage and others by systemic disturbances. In many of the cases the enzymatic defect has not been studied enough, neither is the nature of the metabolic disturbances.

Neuronal lipofuscinosis /Batten Disease/ is such an example; it is a joint clinical term and includes several diseases which in the past were considered to be variants of Tay-Sachs Disease. The enzymatic defect responsible for them has not been discovered yet. It is established only that probably there is accumulation of lipofuscin-like substance in nerve cells. The disorders in this group are classified according to their clinical manifestations, morphologic changes and onset, namely: early infantile form, late infantile form, juvenile form, late form.

5.1. Early Infantile Form.

Its course does not differ significantly from the one of Tay-Sachs Disease.

5.2. Late Infantile Form /Jansku-Bielschowsky Type/.

It occurs between the 2nd and 5th year of childhood.

Diffuse cerebral atrophy is seen morphologically, with more marked changes in the granular layer of the cerebellum. There is extensive accumulation of sudanophil and PAS-positive substance in the cytoplasm of neurons, which are ballooned and the nuclei are shifted to the periphery. Electron microscopically neurons are filled with various lipofuscin-like structures. Pigment degeneration is observed in the fundi.

Psychomotor delay with progressing weakening of vision is characteristic of the clinical course. Cerebellar manifestations are typical: ataxias, nystagmus, etc. Quadripareses and epileptic seizures may be observed. Patients die within 3-4 years with manifestations of cachexia and bulbar paralysis.

5.3. Juvenile Form /Spielmeyer-Vogt Type/.

The disease begins at the age of 7-10 years and follows a protracted course.

Morphologic changes are not different from those in the late infantile form. Inclusions in the form of fine, twisted membranes and massive accumulation of lipofuscin material are seen electron microscopically.

Clinical manifestations. Disturbances of equilibrium and vision are predominant and epileptic seizures are rare. Progressive optic atrophy leads to amblyopia and amaurosis. Severe intellectual degradation develops with disruption of speech. In the terminal stage there is spastic quadriplegia and severe dementia.

5.4. Late Form /Kufs Disease/.

It begins after 10 years of age. Classical pathomorphologic examination does not show any specific changes. Electron microscopy detects cytoplasmic inclusions, containing lipofuscin.

Frequent intense myoclonus involving the whole body, sometimes together with choreoathetosic hyperkinesias is characteristic for the clinical course. Visual fields are narrowed; there is hemeralopia. Dementia manifestations progress and epileptic seizures are not obligatory.

6. Myoclonus epilepsy.

A hereditary degenerative disorder which is characterized by coexistence of grand mal epileptic seizures, myoclonus and severe dementia.

Synonyms. Unvericht disease, Unvericht-Lundborg disease, familial myoclonus, progressive myoclonus epilepsy, progressive familial epilepsy, familial progressive epileptic myoclonus, familial progressive myoclonic epilepsy, Unvericht-Lundborg progressive familial myoclonic epilepsy.

Etiology and pathogenesis. The disorder it transmitted in autosomal recessive pattern. The primary biochemical defect in myoclonus epilepsy is not well understood. A decreased level of mucopolysaccharides in plasma is frequently detected in patients, which is used for early diagnosis of the disease. The level of arginine succinic acid is increased. Disturbance in the metabolism of serotonin and gamma-amino butyric acid is suggested in the pathogenesis.

Pathomorphology. Pathomorphological changes are localized mainly in nucleus dentatus of the cerebellum, substantia nigra, nucleus ruber and anterior cerebellar peduncles. Amyloid-like inclusions in neurons, known as Lafora bodies, are typical. They may be single or multiple. These bodies are complex polyglycoside-protein compounds and may be detected not only in CNS, but also in the liver, spleen, cardiac muscle, skeletal muscles and peripheral nerves.

Clinical manifestations. The disorder usually begins between 6 and 16 years of age. Myoclonic hyperkinesias, grand mal epileptic seizures, progressive dementia and extrapyramidal rigidity are characteristic. Hyperkinesias are of various types. In some patients they are indiscriminate, nonrhythmic and nonsynchronous contractions of individual muscles. In other cases myoclonic jerks are rapid contractions of entire muscle groups. These hyperkinesias are also disorderly, diffuse and nonrhythmic. It is typical for myoclonic jerks to be enhanced by visual, auditory and other sensory stimulants. Myoclonus is also intensified by cold exposure and eye closure. They are less pronounced at rest and disappear during sleep. In most patients myoclonic jerks become more frequent before the seizure and decrease and disappear significantly afterwards. They usually begin in the upper extremities and then spread to the neck, face and trunk. Sometimes they also involve the soft palate, pharynx and diaphragm.

Epileptic seizures usually occur at night in the form of a generalized convulsion with loss of consciousness, loss of sphincter control, tonic and clonic jerks and tongue bite. After completion of the seizure patients are somnolent or fall asleep. Gradually seizures become more frequent; petit mal, complex partial, simple partial seizures and other types of epilepsy may occur.

In the terminal stage of the disease seizures gradually disappear, speech becomes dysarthic, swallowing is impaired. Severe dementia develops. Marasmus and cachexia become evident. Parkinson-like syndrome appears sometimes: muscle rigidity, bradykinesia and bradymimia. In some cases endocrine disturbances are observed: obesity, hirsutism, etc.

EEG investigation shows paroxysmal high-voltage activity enhanced by photostimulation and hyperventilation.

Diagnosis and differential diagnosis. The diagnosis myoclonus epilepsy is made on the basis of the characteristic triad of symptoms: myoclonic hyperkinesias, grand mal epileptic seizures and severe dementia. Differential diagnosis is first made with the types of epilepsy. Appearance of hyperkinesias in strictly determined muscle groups and their continuation during sleep are typical for partial epileptic seizures /Kozevnikov type/. Atrophy and pareses are often noted in these muscle groups. In idiopathic generalized epileptic seizures dementia occurs not before the late stages of the disease and not obligatory. In these cases there is no positive family history. Hunt's myoclonic dyssinergia follows a similar course. Cerebellar symptoms, intention tremor, ataxia, etc. are characteristic of the latter besides hyperkinesias.

Evolution. The disorder may last for 10-20 years, sometimes even longer.

Treatment. Symptomatic and directed towards control of epileptic seizures. Anticonvulsant medications are used: Phenobarbital, Antelepsin, Tegretol, Depakine, etc. Nootropic agents are also applied /Nootropil/, as well as cholinolytic drugs.

Prophylaxis. Genetic counseling.

7. Leukodystrophies.

Leukodystrophies are a rare group of genetic disorders of the nervous system, which are a result of metabolic defects in the formation of myelin. Some authors speak of primary leukodystrophies, which are actually a form of lipidoses caused by a primary genetic defect in the metabolism of myelin and secondary leukodystrophies, i.e. due to disturbances in the metabolism of amino acids caused by other reasons.

Metachromatic leukodystrophy is the most common of this group of disorders.

7.1. Metachromatic Leukodystrophy.

A hereditary disease, in which coordination disturbances, pareses and cognitive delay develop, due to degeneration of myelin in central and peripheral nervous system and accumulation of sulfatides.

Etiology and pathogenesis. The disorder is inherited in autosomal recessive pattern and affects both genders. Deficiency of the enzyme arylsulfatatse A, which takes part in the metabolism of sulfatides, lies in the basis of the pathogenesis. As a result of this there is accumulation of galactosyl 3-sulfate ceramide in myelin /39, 62/.

Pathomorphology. Accumulation of sulfatides in stellate reticuloendothelial cells of the liver and renal tubules is found pathomorphologically. Ganglial cells of the retina might also be affected. The brain shows marked congestion of the white matter.

Diffuse demyelinization, glial proliferation and metachromatic inclusions in cells, which give the name of the disorder, are typical.

Clinical manifestations. The symptoms of the disease appear at 2-3 years of age and sometimes earlier. It begins with progressive weakness in the legs and muscle hypotonia, but spasticity can also be observed. Atactic manifestations progress, vision gradually declines, dementia and loss of acquired skills occur. In the beginning tendon reflexes are decreased and later they become pathologically increased. In approximately half of the patients epileptic seizures appear. In the late stages of the disease vision and hearing are severely impaired, manifestations of bulbar paralysis are evident, decerebration rigidity increases, cachexia occurs /17/.

Diagnosis and differential diagnosis. Antenatal diagnosis is made by measuring the enzyme activity in cultured fibroblasts, isolated lymphocytes, serum or urine. A biopsy of a peripheral nerve /most often the sural nerve/ is performed, the activity of the enzyme arylsulfatase is measured in urine, or metachromatic bodies are searched for microscopically in urine. There is protein cell dissociation in CSF. CSF protein reaches up to 1-2 g/l. The concentration of sulfatides is increased in plasma, CSF, urine and biopsy specimen.

Differential diagnosis is made with other leukodystrophies and with lipidoses.

Evolution. The course of the disease is progressive. Lethal outcome occurs in 2-3 years. Rarely patients survive until 10 years of age.

Treatment. No specific therapy exists. A diet with a low content of vitamin A is prescribed. If there are epileptic seizures, anticonvulsive and other symptomatic agents are used.

Prophylaxis. Adequate genetic counseling, finding heterozygous carriers and antenatal diagnosis are of great importance.

7.2. Orthochromatic Leukodystrophy.

Synonyms. Late form of sudanophil leukodystrophy, sudanophil leukodystrophy.

Etiology and pathogenesis. The disorder is inherited in autosomal recessive pattern.

Pathomorphology. Pathomorphologically the brain is atrophic, with diffuse demyelinization and marked gliosis. Orthochromatic, slightly sudanophil and PAS-negative lipofuscin-like substance is found histologically. The concentration of cholesterol might be increased. Disturbed myelin metabolism is probably the major pathogenetic mechanism here, similar to metachromatic leukodystrophy. There exists a separate form of the disease where atrophy of adrenal cortex is present concurrently with the changes in the brain.

Clinical manifestations. The disorder is characterized clinically by cerebellar symptoms, dementia and involvement of the pyramidal tracts in the form of pareses. Blindness also occurs during the late stages. When adrenal glands are affected, symptoms of Addison's disease are apparent and they may precede neurologic symptoms.

Treatment. Symptomatic. In case of adrenal insufficiency, appropriate hormonal therapy is given.

7.3. Rare Forms of Leukodystrophies.

7.3.1. Globoid Cell Leukodystrophy.

Synonyms. Krabbe globoid cell dystrophy, Krabbe disease, galactosylceramide lipidosis, progressive cerebral polydystrophy in small children.

Etiology and pathogenesis. A defect in the metabolism of the enzyme galactoside-ceramide-β-galactosidase in brain tissue, spleen and liver is inherited in autosomal recessive pattern.

Pathomorphology. The brain is atrophic, and the white matter is of very dense consistency. Diffuse demyelinization is found with preservation only of U-fibers and massive loss of oligodendroglial cells. Globoid cells /which gave the name of the disease/ are found single or in groups around small vessels. Deposits of galactocerebrosides and enlargement of cytoplasmic structures are detected electron microscopically in Schwann cells of peripheral nervous system and histiocytes of endoneural space. Straight or convoluted tubules with irregular crystalloid cross section or tubular profiles similar to those in Gaucher disease are also found.

Clinical manifestations. The following forms are distinguished: congenital, infantile, juvenile and in adults. The disease develops more frequently in boys at the age of 3-4 months. There is arrest in motor development, increased irritability, convulsions and muscle hypertonia. Optic atrophy, hearing impairment, cachexia, decerebration rigidity and quadriparesis are later added to these symptoms. Increased protein concentration is found in CSF.

Treatment. Symptomatic. It includes mostly anticonvulsants and tranquilizers.

7.3.2. Peliceaus-Merzbacher Disease.

Synonyms. Infantile chronic diffuse sclerosis, familial centrolobular sclerosis, aplasia axialis extracorticalis congenital.

Etiology and pathogenesis. The pathologic gene is recessive and it is localized in X-chromosome because of which mainly boys suffer from the disease.

Pathomorphology. Diffuse demyelinization of white matter is found, which is preserved in small islets only around vessels. Axons are relatively preserved ; there are deposits of orthochromatic, sudanophil substances.

Clinical manifestations. Initial manifestations appear during the first year of life, around the 3rd-4th month. Children are floppy, hypotonic; ataxia, intentional tremor and choreoathetosic hyperkinesias develop. Spastic para- and quadripareses, extrapyramidal rigidity and Parkinsonism manifestations are added gradually. Optic atrophy and progressive intellectual decline develop.

Evolution. The disorder progresses slowly. There are patients who have reached 50 years of age. Sometimes short remissions are observed.

There are two most common clinico-morphological variants of the disease:

a/ Seitelberger leukodystrophy. It is a congenital variant of the disorder. Its course, however, is more rapid. No significant differences are found morphologically with the exception of some additional malformations, i.e. microgyria.

b/ Zöwenberg-Hell leukodystrophy. It occurs more often in adulthood and the leading presentation is psychotic signs and not intellectual decline. In some instances, however, it affects children as well: microcephals or dwarfs.

7.4. Leukodystrophies with Secondary disturbance of Myelin Metabolism and Structure.

7.4.1. Aminoacidurias.

With the term aminoacidurias are designated metabolic disturbances in the pathways of amino acids. There are two types of them: primary and secondary.

In primary aminoacidurias there is increased excretion of one or more amino acids in urine. The latter may also be increased in blood, CSF, sweat and bowel secretions. The elevated level of amino acids is caused by a genetic defect in the enzymes carrying out their metabolism. Secondary aminoacidurias are observed in some systemic diseases such as hepatolenticular degeneration, renal disorders, rickets, etc.

The clinical course of aminoacidurias is similar and their differentiation is accomplished with the aid of specific biochemical tests.

7.4.2. Phenylketonuria.

A hereditary degenerative disorder of the nervous system, which develops as a result of an enzyme defect in the metabolism of amino acids and is characterized by pyramidal signs, seizures and mental retardation.

Frequency. It is most prevalent in Scandinavian countries and is very rare among African people. 1 child with phenylketonuria is born to approximately 15 000 births.

Etiology and pathogenesis. It is transmitted in autosomal recessive pattern. It is caused by deficiency of the enzyme phenylalanine hydroxylase because of which phenylalanine cannot turn into tyrosine. As a result the level of phenylalanine in plasma increases and reaches up to 900 µmol/l. the accumulation of phenylalanine leads to irreversible brain damage. There is impaired myelinization, neurotransmitter pathways, metabolism of nucleic acids, proteins and fats.

Pathomorphology. Demyelinization and gliosis are detected in CNS. Cystic degeneration in white and grey matter develops.

Clinical manifestations. The major symptom of the disease is delayed mental development at a various degree. Periods of improvement are observed in some children: smiling, eye traction. After some time, however, these functions disappear again. Grand mal and petit mal seizures occur often, usually during the second half of the first year of life. Motor disturbances in the early stage of the disease are characterized by decreased muscle tone. Dystonia and muscle hypertonia develop later. Tendon reflexes are pathologically increased, with increased reflexogenic areas; clonus, coordination disturbances and hyperkinesias may be observed. Children learn to walk later, the gait is spastic-atactic; speech is disturbed. With advance of the disease schizophrenic languorous behavior is observed. The patients' outer appearance is characteristic: the children are with blond hair, blue eyes, skin pigmentation is disturbed. Exudative diathesis, dermatitis, eczema, etc. develop frequently. The specific "mousy" odor is characteristic.

Diagnosis and differential diagnosis. Detection of high concentration of phenylalanine in plasma and phenylpyruvic acid in urine is important for the diagnosis of phenylketonuria. As differential diagnosis one should have in mind other amino acid metabolism disorders in childhood, sequelae of birth trauma and asphyxia, as well as infections of CNS.

Evolution. The disorder progresses slowly. In case of adequate treatment the prognosis is favorable. Untreated patients develop severe mental handicap.

Treatment. Dietary treatment is most important. High-protein products – meat, eggs, cheese, walnuts, etc. – must be almost completely excluded from the patients' diet, and foods rich in iron and vitamins must be increased. On the other hand phenylalanine is an essential amino acid and the body should not be entirely deprived of it. Its intake is calculated on an individual basis and is around 40-

80 mg/kg. Plasma phenylalanine should be kept ata level of 300-485 μmol/l. Treatment is conducted up to 12-14 years of age; afterwards low-protein intake is enough for well-being.

Prophylaxis. Heterozygous carriers of the pathologic gene are detected with the aid of a loading test with phenylalanine. Their prevalence in population is at the rate of 1:50-1:70. Phenylalanine concentration in amniotic fluid is also measured.

8. Other Metabolic Disturbances Affecting the Nervous System.

8.1. Syndromes in Disturbed Cholesterol Metabolism.

Several diseases are included here, in which disturbances in cholesterol metabolism lead to accumulation of lipids in the nervous system, bones and internal organs.

8.1.1. Hand-Schüller-Cristian Disease.

Synonyms. Schüller-Christian syndrome, Christian syndrome, cholesterine disease, cholesterine lipidosis, cranial pituitary granulomatosis, xanthomatous reticulo-endotheliosis, systemic xanthogranulomatosis, dysostosis craniohypophysaria, xanthomatosis craniohypophysaria, reticuloendotheliosis craniohypophysaria.

Etiology and pathogenesis. It is not known for certain whether the disorder is a redult of primary disturbance if lipid metabolism or a generalized granulomatosis with secondary cholesterol deposition in tissues. Dominant inheritance with reduced penetrance in regard to lipid metabolism is assumed.

Pathomorphology. Granulomatose infiltrates of meninges and nerve roots and massive intracerebral nodular structures are found. In other cases there are scattered microgranulomas in brain tissue, with subsequent demyelinization. Reticulo-histiocytes proliferate and are filled with cholesterol /xanthomatous foamy cells/. Granulomatose expansion affects cranial pituitary area, internal organs and bones.

Clinical manifestations. It usually begins in early childhood but may affect any age. Endocrine disturbances are the leading clinical manifestations due to the localization: pituitary nanism and infantilism, diabetes insipidus, adipose-genital dystrophy, obesity and cachexia, glycosuria, exophthalmus. On the side of the nervous system, scattered pyramidal symptoms are often observed, resembling disseminated sclerosis, cranial nerve involvement / often deafness/, sometimes meningeal signs, neuralgic pain, etc. In approximately half of the patients hepatosplenomegaly and skin changes are found.

Roentgenologic examination shows bone lacunas in cranial bones.

The prognosis is poor, particularly when the disorder has begun in early childhood.

Treatment is symptomatic and is directed to lowering cholesterol level.

8.1.2. L. Van Bogaert Cerebrotendinous Xanthomatosis.

Etiology and pathogenesis. The disorder is assumed to be inherited in autososmal recessive pattern. It occurs in siblings.

Pathomorphology. The disease is characterized by marked demyelinization in the cerebellum and brain stem, with deposition of cholesterol in them. Tumor-like deposits, containing cholesterol and phosphatides are found on Achilles tendons.

Clinical manifestations. The disease is characterized clinically by cerebellar signs, pyramidal symptoms, myoclonic jerks, seizure disorders and deafness. Patients' mental development is delayed /30/.

The course is progressive. The prognosis is poor.

8.2. Syndromes of Disturbed Pyrine Metabolism.

8.2.1. Lesch-Nyhan Syndrome.

This is a type of hyperuricemia caused by deficiency of the enzyme hypoxanthine-guanine phosphoribosyltran sferase /HGPRT/.

Synonyms. Congenital hyperuricemia with mental retardation, athetosis and self-injuries.

Etiology and pathogenesis. It is inherited in X-recessive pattern. Boys are affected and females are asymptomatic carriers.

There are enzyme variants. Congenital deficiency of HGPRT leads to disturbed purine metabolism with excessive increase of uric acid in the nervous system and some organs. Symptoms result from the toxic effect of uric acid on them.

Pathomorphology. Diffuse demyelinization in cerebral hemispheres and cerebellum, in the granular layer of which there is degeneration.

Clinical manifestations. The manifestations appear at approximately 1 year of age: children stop eating well, learn to walk later. Progressive choreoathetosis, spastic rigidity, opisthotonus, pathologically increased reflexes, quadriparesis occur afterwards. Mental retardation is accompanied by behavioral changes and tendency for autoaggression: self-eating of lips and fingers is typical, despite preserved pain sensitivity. Subcutaneous urate nodules are formed and gouty arthritis develops later. Renal calculosis with hematuria develops in most patients.

Diagnosis and differential diagnosis. The diagnosis is made on the basis of clinical signs and biochemical tests: hyperuricemia above 535 μmol/l, hyperuricuria, the ratio (uric acid/creatinine) is 3.0 with a reference value of 1.5 in newborns and 0.6 in 10-year olds. The activity of HGPRT is measured in fibroblasts, hair follicles and erythrocytes. Differential diagnosis is made with gout, leucosis, increased excretion of uric acid in tubular defects caused by some drugs. Hyperuricemia may also be observed with alcoholism, hyperlipoproteinemia type III, glycogenosis type I, etc.

Evolution. The course is slow, progressive, with a poor prognosis.

Treatment. Allopurinol, L-DOPA and 5-hydroxytryptophan are used to improve cerebral disturbances.

Prophylaxis. Genetic counseling. Antenatal investigation of amniotic cells is performed. Disease carriers are also examined.

Chapter V

SYSTEMIC ATROPHIES OF CORTICOSPINAL AND CORTICOBULBAR MOTOR NEURON SYSTEMS

Degenerative disorders of the nervous system affecting motor tracts and neurons are known under the joint name Motor System Disease. This term includes progressive atrophic changes in motor neurons of the cortex, brain stem and spinal cord, where clinical signs of damage to the corticospinal and corticobulbar tracts are observed. Amyotrophic Lateral Sclerosis /LAS/ is a typical representative of this group of disorders.

1. Amyotrophic Lateral Sclerosis.

A chronic progressive disease of the nervous system, characterized by damage to the

motor neurons of the cerebrum and spinal cord, degeneration of the corticospinal and corticobulbar fibers.

Frequency. In most cases the disorder is sporadic; it occurs at an incidence of 0.4-1.76/100 000 people. Families affected by the disease are also encountered.

Etiology and pathogenesis. Not well understood. It is considered that constitutional and exogenous /mainly infectious/ factors combine in most cases. Hereditary predisposition is also important /80/. There are case reports of affected people in several generations, and also among siblings. Some authors regard the disorder as a manifestation of slow virus infection. This presumption is based on a series of experimental animal models. The test animals are infected with emulsion of dead patients' brains and as a result clinical and morphological features similar to ALS develop. There exists a hypothesis according to which combination of constitutional hereditary predisposition and neurotropic "slow" viruses is necessary for the development of ALS. Previously impaired immunity /influenza, arboviruses, enteroviruses, etc./ is usually a condition needed for manifestation of slow virus infections. Risk factors con also be protein, vitamin or microelement deficiency, as well as disorders of the gastrointestinal tract. Predisposing factors in adults can also be some vascular disease of the nervous system, predominantly vertebrobasilar insufficiency.

The pathogenesis of the disorder is determined mainly by disturbances in the metabolism of proteins, amino acids and carbohydrates. This is confirmed by decreased total protein and arginine plasma level and elevated globulins /especially in the bulbar form of the disease/, tyrosine, histidine and serine. There is increased excretion of valine, leucine, arginine in urine.

Pathomorphology. Degenerative changes are found mostly in the region of the cervical intumescence and the anterior horns of the spinal cord, the lateral columns, the brain stem – the nuclei of V, VII, IX, X, XI and XII cranial nerves, the reticular formation, the cerebral cortex – in the cells of gyrus centralis anterior and posterior /mainly in layer III and IV/ and in the pyramidal tracts. A significant portion of the preserved neurons are small, wrinkled and filled with lipofuscin. Astrocytes proliferate in the place of dead neurons. Subcortical nuclei and the cerebellum, autonomic centers in the spinal cord, rubrothalamic and rubrospinal tracts, blood vessels of the cerebellum and spinal cord are less affected. The walls of these vessels are thickened, with lymphocytic infiltrates around them. Oxyphil cytoplasmic inclusions are often found in motoneurons of the spinal cord and medulla oblongata.

Clinical manifestations. They are determined by symptoms of upper and lower motor neuron damage. Finger movements are gradually impaired, they become clumsy and muscle power decreases. Muscle atrophies and pareses of distal parts of the upper extremities accompanied by fibrillations and fasciculations develop within a few weeks or months. The latter are usually symmetric, affecting muscles of the shoulder girdle, back and chest. Atrophies are most prominent in the small muscles of the fingers and wrists and fingers gradually become like "bird claws" and the hand resembles a "monkey paw".

From the leg muscles those responsible for dorsal flexion of the foot are more frequently affected, and from bulbar muscles those of the tongue and soft palate are electively damaged. Extensors are more severely affected than flexors. Diffuse muscle atrophy is observed significantly more rarely. In case of predominant involvement of the spinal cord patients later die of respiratory disturbances of spinal origin. If lower motor neuron damage prevails, tendon and periostal reflexes are decreased.

Another characteristic of ALS is pyramidal symptomatics / due to involvement of the upper motor neuron/. It presents clinically with muscle hypertonia, especially in the lower extremities, abnormally increased reflexes and presence of pathologic reflexes from Babinski and Rossolimo group. Generally these changes are relatively constant and are observed for the four extremities. Spontaneous jaw clonus and trismus are not rare. As atrophies progress, spasticity decreases and may even disappear, but hyperreflexia persists. Intensified mandibular reflex is typical for ALS and is seen in almost all patients. Oral automatisms are also very frequent. Symptoms of damage to subcortical nuclei are rarely encountered. Involvement of the nuclei of the cranial nerves in the brain stem is characteristic of ALS. Disturbances in phonation, articulation and swallowing: dysphonia, dysarthria and dysphagia, develop and increase gradually. Tongue movements are limited; it is atrophic, with fibrillations. The soft palate droops, the pharyngeal reflex disappears, patients choke while swallowing. Mimic muscles are subsequently affected. The face becomes amimic, the mandible droops, chewing becomes difficult due to damage to the Vth and VIIth cranial nerves. Bilateral involvement of corticobulbar tracts results in pseudobulbar paralysis: oral automatisms, involuntary cry and laughter /76/. Besides skeletal muscles other systems are also affected by the pathological process: gastrointestinal dyskinesias are observed, myocardial contractility is decreased. Generally sensitivity is not changed, except in some rare cases. The brain stem is involved in terminal stages of the disease and patients die of severe respiratory and heart failure /72/.

There are 4 major clinical forms of ALS according to localization: high, bulbar, cervicothoracic and lumbosacral. In patients with the high form of the disease symptoms of damage to the pyramidal tracts prevail: spastic quadripareses, symptoms of involvement of the anterior spinal horns and mental events of variable degree. In the bulbar form the pathologic process is localized predominantly in the brain stem. Severe respiratory and swallowing disturbances with preserved motor activity are leading in these patients. Amyotrophic pareses of the arms and spastic pareses of the legs are characteristic for the cervicothoracic form. In the lumbosacral form there are amyotrophic pareses in the lower limbs and moderate pyramidal symptomatics.

Diagnosis and differential diagnosis. International criteria for diagnosing ALS have been established. They include the following:

1/ Clinical evidence of lower motor neuron degeneration by neuropathologic or electrophysiological examination,

2/ Clinical evidence of upper motor neuron degeneration by clinical examination.

3/ Progressive spread of these symptoms from one region to other regions.

Further diagnostic criteria include the absence of:

1/ Electrophysiological evidence of other disease processes that might explain the signs of upper motor neuron /UMN/ and lower motor neuron /LMN/ degeneration.

2/ Neuroimaging /roentgenologic, CT and MRI/ evidence of other disease processes that might explain the observed clinical and electrophysiological signs.

Studies used to confirm the diagnosis of ALS.

EMG changes in 2 or more muscles, innervated by LMN from 2 or more regions: bulbar, cervical, thoracic or lumbosacral are of great importance.

LMN degeneration is present in case of:

a/ reduced EMG recording;

b/ presence of high-voltage axion potentials;

c/ reduction in fibrillar potentials;

There is probable LMN degeneration in case of:

a/ reduced EMG recording;

b/ reduction in the motor units with registration of macropotentials;

There is possible LMN degeneration in case of:

a/ reduced EMG recording with polyphasic potentials of low amplitude;

b/ decreased conduction velocity by over 30%;

c/ absence of fasciculations;

Electrophysiological evidence of UMN degeneration is:

a/ Decreased conduction velocity of UMN by over 30%;

b/ Decreased amplitude of SEP by more than 10%.

Neuroimaging techniques /roentgenograms, CT and MRI/ do not demonstrate ALS-specific changes. Laboratory tests are also nonspecific. Sometimes /in approximately 20% of cases/ there is mild elevation of CSF protein with no changes in globulin fractions /23/. Pathomorphologic studies of a biopsy specimen from a muscle or peripheral nerve show evidence of a degenerative process with no specific changes.

Based on the diagnostic investigations and electrophysiological findings there are:

1/ Clinically Definite ALS: in the presence of symptoms of UMN and LMN degeneration from the bulbar region or symptoms or UMN and LMN degeneration in at least two regions. There are no electrophysiological, roentgenologic or laboratory changes which is of great importance.

2/ Clinically Probable ALS: in the presence of clinical evidence alone by UMN and LMN signs in at least two regions. Various combinations of symptoms from UMN and LMN are possible.

3/ Clinically Possible ALS: when clinical signs of UMN and LMN dysfunction are found together in only one region or UMN signs are found alone in two or more regions; or LMN signs are found rostral to UMN signs.

4/ Clinically Suspected ALS: when there are clinical signs of LMN dysfunction in two or more regions. Indirect signs of UMN dysfunction might be discovered by additional investigations.

Differential diagnosis is first made with ALS-mimic syndromes. They can be observed in the following cases: hematologic disorders /Waldenström's disease, myeloma, lymphomas, etc./, endocrinopathies /hyperthyroidism, hyperparathyroidism/, cancer of the lungs, colon, etc., vasculites, exogenous poisoning /with lead, mercury, arsenic, pesticides/, severe deforming spondylosis, etc. In the early stages of ALS differential diagnosis with several diseases has to be made. First one should consider multiple sclerosis and mainly its forms involving predominantly the brain stem and the spinal cord. The presence of Bauer's criteria for disseminated sclerosis makes the diagnosis easier. Viral encephalitis is distinguished from ALS based on the history of an acute disease onset, epidemiologic situation, CSF changes and its more favorable course. Subacute anterior poliomyelitis ascends with gradual involvement of motor neurons in the spinal cord and brain stem. Here bulbar symptoms and atrophies are present as well, but there are no pyramidal signs. In the later stages the disease must be distinguished first from vertebrogenic cervical myelopathy. Its course is generally benign with local segmental symptomatics and disturbed sensation in the arms. Nerve root pain, pelvic reservoir dysfunction and asymmetric paralyses are present. Roentgenogram of cervical vertebra shows marked osteochondrosis. EMG is negative. Progressive bulbar paralysis differs from ALS by its relatively slower progression of symptoms and by its usually normal mandibular reflex. Intramedullar tumors are differentiated from ALS mostly with the aid of some contrast roentgenologic techniques: myelography, magnetic resonance imaging, and by the high level of CSF protein, etc. Syringomyelia, which also presents with distal atrophies, is characterized by long duration, pain syndrome, syringomyelic sensory deficit, vasomotor and trophic disturbances and dysraphic changes. ALS is distinguished from Creutzfeldt-Jacob Disease by the absence of prominent mental and extrapyramidal signs. Chronic progressive spinal atrophy in adults /Aran-Duchenne form/is characterized by descending symptoms: atrophies begin in the muscles of the wrists and shoulders and spread towards the legs. In this case again there are no pyramidal signs. Progressive proximal muscle atrophy /Kugelberg-Welander/ differs with gradually increasing weakness, atrophies and fasciculations in proximal parts of the trunk and extremities. The disease resembles not only ALS, but also a myopathy: recessive pattern of inheritance, onset in adolescence, slow progression, pseudohypertrophy and absence of bulbar symptoms.

Evolution. The course of the disorder is slow, progressive. Patients die of somatic complications within 2.5-10 years.

Treatment. There is no specific medication. Metabolism stimulating agents are indicated: vitamins B, vitamin E, ATP, Nootropil, Cerebrolysin, anabolic drugs are indicated. Thyrotropin-releasing hormone in small doses subcutaneously or intramuscularly is also used. Gangliosides, Interferon, guanidine hydrochlorides, the experimental drug Risolym are also prescribed. Application of Nivalin, Dibazol, etc. is indicated for improvement of neuromuscular conduction. Spasticity is reduced by Baclofen, Scutamil, Mydocalm. With development of bulbar symptoms, patients are fed via nasogastric tube and life-saving procedures are undertaken /54/.

Prophylaxis. Prophylaxis is not well studied. Probably physiologic pregnancy, prevention of infections, intoxications and birth trauma could decrease the risk of developing the disorder. Secondary prophylaxis includes foundation of ALS-patients' associations where the nature of the disease course is being explained, as well as the ways of caring for the patients and the emergency measures in case of development of bulbar symptoms.

2. Progressive Bulbar Paralysis. Fazio-Londe Syndrome.

A hereditary degenerative or sporadic disease, characterized by clinical signs of
involvement of caudal cranial nerves which progresses.

Synonyms. Progressive familial bulbar paralysis in children.

Etiology and pathogenesis. Not well understood. There are reports of quite a few familial cases of developing the disease which point to autosomal recessive pattern of inheritance, as well as of sporadic cases.

Pathomorphology. Prominent lesions in the anterior horn cells of the spinal cord and in the nuclei of the caudal cranial nerves are found. Anterior roots are also affected. neurogenic atrophy, identical to that in Werdnig-Hoffman disease, is seen in skeletal muscles.

Clinical manifestations. The disease begins near the end of the second year of life when bulbar symptoms develop: dysarthria, dysphagia and dysphonia, paresis of the abducens nerve, respiratory disturbance and weakness of the facial muscles. Tongue atrophy is frequently observed. Sometimes the nerves that control eye movement and the motor part of the trigeminal nerve are affected. In other cases peripheral pareses or paralyses of the limbs are added to the bulbar disturbances, as a sign of pyramidal disturbance and facial nerve paralysis.

Diagnosis and differential diagnosis. The diagnosis is made on the basis of the clinical course and the pathomorphological changes. As a differential diagnosis one should have in mind the following: Duchenne syndrome, myasthenia gravis, Guillain-Barré polyradiculoneuritis, Oppenheim's myatonia, brain stem tumors and the bulbar form of poliomyelitis.

Evolution. The disease progresses rapidly. Death occurs in 6-12 months following the presentation of the initial signs.

Treatment. Symptomatic. It is directed to management of bulbar symptoms.

Prophylaxis. There are no effective prophylactic measures.

3. Strümpell Disease.

A chronic progressive hereditary degenerative disorder of the nervous system which is
characterized by bilateral involvement of the pyramidal tracts in the spinal cord.

Synonyms. Strümpell's familial spastic paralysis, Erb-Charcot-_Strümpell's familial spastic paralysis.

Etiology and pathogenesis. The disease is transmitted in autosomal dominant or autosomal recessive pattern. In the first case its course is more severe. The pure forms of familial spastic paraplegia are more often inherited in a dominant pattern. The pathogenesis of the degenerative process and the primary biochemical defect are not known /44/.

Pathomorphology. The damage to the lumbar and thoracic part of the spinal cord are most severe; the brain stem and sometimes the cerebral cortex are less affected. Glial changes in the pyramidal tracts in the lateral columns of the spinal cord are found, and similar changes in its anterior columns, spinocerebellar tracts and posterior columns where they are less prominent. There is degeneration and neuronal death in the region of the anterior central gyrus /layer III and V/, Purkinje cells in the cerebellum, in the motoneurons in the brain stem and the spinal cord.

Clinical manifestations. The disorder develops gradually. Most often the initial symptoms present during the second decade of life, but variations in the age of onset are possible between 13 and 30 years of age and even later. In the beginning there is stiffness in the legs while moving, increased tiredness and difficulties in motion. The objective neurologic examination in the early stages of the disease reveals spastic paraparesis of the legs with increased muscle tone, abnormally increased reflexes and pathological reflexes from the Babinski and Rossolimo group, clonus of the patella and the foot. The gait becomes spastic – paraparetic – the foot deforms and "Friedreich's foot" is observed. Joint contractures and deformities may be seen. Superficial reflexes are usually not affected, there is no sensory or pelvic reservoir impairment, coordination is preserved, intellect also. The arms are involved considerably later and not in all cases. The muscle tone in the upper extremities is increased, tendon and periostal reflexes are increased, pathologic reflexes appear also. Pseudobulbar symptoms are frequent. Spacticity prevails over the paresis. In most cases along with spastic paraparesis of the legs there are symptoms of damage to other systems: scandic speech, palpebral ptosis, optic atrophy, nystagmus and intention tremor, distal muscle atrophies, etc. Clinical symptoms, characteristic of both familial spastic paraplegia and Friedreich's and Pierre Marie's disease, are often seen. Transition forms between these disorders have been reported, as well as between Strümpell Disease and amyotrophic syndromes. All of this indicates pronounced clinical polymorphism of this disorder.

Diagnosis and differential diagnosis. The diagnosis is usually not very difficult to establish given a positive family history and the characteristic clinical manifestations of the disease. EMG is useful in the early diagnostics; it demonstrates rhythmic, scattered, low-amplitude biopotentials type II of the lower extremities. Examination of the CSF shows no pathological changes.

In atypical sporadic forms the disorder must be distinguished from several diseases following a similar course. The spinal form of multiple sclerosis has a number of other characteristics along with spastic paraparesis of the legs: a remitting course, impermanent presentation and fading of the individual symptoms, pelvic reservoir impairment, disappearance of the abdominal superficial reflexes, CSF changes, etc., absence of positive family history. In contrast to ALS, Strümpell Disease begins at an earlier age, the lower motor neuron is not affected /there are no fasciculations, atrophy of the small muscles of the wrist, degeneration reaction on the EMG/., there are no bulbar symptoms. Segmental sensory disturbances, asymmetric damage to the extremities and impaired CSF circulation, demonstrated by the syndrome of protein-cell dissociation, are important in distinguishing the disorder from extramedullar tumors and spinal cord compression syndrome caused by various factors. Different from Strümpell Disease, in neurolues the typical rash is observed, as well as symptoms of involvement of the posterior columns, characteristic visual disturbances and blood and CSF changes at serologic investigation. Other degenerative disorders of the nervous system should be kept in mind, Little's disease in the first place, which is characterized by presentation soon after birth, lack of progression of the symptoms and considerably more favorable course.

Evolution. The disease shows slow progression. Its course is more unfavorable if it begins at an early age. In cases of late development of the disorder hypertonia and hyperreflexia prevail over motor disturbances. The prognosis is favorable as for patients' life.

Treatment. Symptomatic. Drugs that decrease muscle tone are prescribed: Mydocalm, Baclofen, Scutamil. Tranquilizers are also used: Seduxen, Tazepam, Elenium. Physiotherapeutic procedures, remedial gym, nootropic agents, vitamins, etc. are applied as well.

Prophylaxis. Genetic counseling.

Chapter VI

HEREDITARY DEGENERATIVE
DISEASES
OF SPINAL MOTONEURONS

1. Spinal Muscular Atrophies.

Spinal muscular atrophies are hereditary degenerative diseases, predominantly autosomal recessive, in which degenerative processes affect anterior horn cells of the spinal cord and possibly motor nuclei of cranial nerves. In these cases the only structures affected are those of the lower motoneuron, due to which the cardinal clinical features are peripheral pareses, muscle hypotonia, decreased to absent tendon reflexes, etc. Because there are autonomic nerve fibers in anterior nerve roots, sweat secretion and vasomotor disturbances are not rare. The clinical course is quite variable.

Depending on the age of presentation, the affected muscle groups and the clinical course, spinal muscular atrophies are divided into several forms.

I.1. Infantile Form of Werdnig-Hoffmann.

A severe, progressive disease, which develops in early childhood, the main symptoms of which are: weakness and atrophy of the axial muscles and proximal limb muscles.

Synonyms: Severe spinal muscular atrophy of Werdnig-Hoffmann, progressive spinal amyotrophy, spinal muscular atrophy type I.

Frequency. The incidence of the disease is 1:100 000 of the population and 7:100 000 of newborns.

Etiology and pathogenesis. It is inherited mainly in autosomal recessive pattern. High incidence of consanguinity among patients' parents is reported.

Pathology. Marked reduction in the number of neurons it the anterior horns of the spinal cord is observed with severe degeneration in them. In the remaining neurons there is decrease of Nissel substance together with glial expansion. Secondary degeneration of the anterior roots and peripheral nerves also develop, as well as atrophy and degeneration in the motor nuclei in the pons and medulla oblongata, and sometimes in the thalamus and cerebellum. The muscle fibers are thinner and atrophic. Predominantly fibers of histochemical type I are affected, which normally have high oxidase and succinyl dehydrogenase activity, low phosphorylase activity and small quantity of glycogen; muscle fibers type II are insignificantly affected.

Clinical manifestation: There are three main forms of the disease according to the age of manifestation of the first symptoms and the rate of progression – congenital, severe infantile and late form /65/.

In the congenital form there are flaccid fetal movements during late pregnancy in some cases. Typically the children are born with peripheral paralyses affecting proximal limb muscles, sometimes distal muscles as well, muscle, hypotonia, tendon areflexia. Bulbar disturbances are early presented: they include sucking difficulties, tongue fibrillations, decreased pharyngeal reflex. Reduced spontaneous movements are noted: the legs are extended, rotated outwards and lying flat on surfaces - "frog-leg posture". Toddlers fall ahead while sitting. There are often various bone deformities: thin and atrophic fingers, with outstretched hands, high shoulders. Scoliosis, pectus carinatus and joint contractures are present in many children. Intellectual decline is observed in a lot of patients. Developmental anomalies and malformations are encountered in a number of cases: congenital hydrocephalus, cryptorchidism, coxal dysplasia, etc. /66/.

The evolution is rapid, progressive and malignant. Death occurs no later than the age of 5 – 6 years, mostly between 1 – 1.5 years of age. The children die mainly of somatic complications:

cardiovascular failure, pneumonias and respiratory failure because of the weakness of the respiratory muscles and development of bulbar palsy.

In the severe infantile form the first symptoms of the disease present during the second half of the first year of life. Motor skills develop normally in the beginning. The children exhibit good head control and are able to sit. Development of the disease is provoked by infections and intoxications. The child becomes unstable and falls while trying to sit. Gradually all motor skills are lost. The flaccid paralyses, involving the lower extremities, are gradually affecting the arms also. Muscle hypotonia progresses and tendon reflexes disappear. Muscle atrophies, high-frequency tremor of the fingers, tongue fibrillations and muscle contractures occur. In the terminal stages of the disease generalized muscle hypotonia and bulbar palsy develop. Mental development is generally normal.

The course of the severe infantile form is uniformly progressive, though slower compared to the congenital form. Children die of intercurrent infections by the age of 14 – 15 years.

The late form presents around the age of 1.5 – 2 years when motor skills are already developed. It is provoked by trauma and infectious diseases. The progression is gradual. Movements become unstable, with faltering steps, the children often stumble and fall, and get tired while running. A "duck gait" appears. Initially flaccid paralyses spread over proximal muscles of the lower limbs and later over the axial and the upper extremities muscles as well. Typical for this form of the disease are fibrillations and fasciculations of the tongue, bulbar symptoms, tremor of the fingers and decreased pharyngeal reflex. Tendon and periostal reflexes of the extremities disappear early. Bone and joint deformities develop, mainly of the thorax /47/.

The course is more favorable compared to the other forms. The children remain ambulatory until the age of 12 years and die of somatic complication around the age of 20 – 30 years.

Diagnosis and differential diagnosis. The diagnosis is based on the data from a genealogical analysis, confirming autosomal recessive inheritance and the clinical features (early onset, diffuse atrophy predominantly affecting proximal muscles, marked muscle hypotonia, fibrillations and fasciculations and malignant course). EMG shows neurogenic changes, frequent fibrillations, synchronized potentials of fasciculations. In tonic reactions (e.g. while crying) electrical activity increases. ECG shows normal parameters. Muscle biopsy demonstrates typical morphology of the disease. Roentgenograms of long bones show narrowing of the cortical layer and atrophic changes in the epiphyses. Congenital and severe infantile form must be distinguished from congenital muscle hypotonia syndromes. "Floppy infant" syndrome must be considered first. This syndrome may be seen in a number of diseases such as congenital muscular dystrophy, rickets, atonic cerebral palsy, glycogenosis type II, etc. Typical EMG evidence of anterior horn damage confirms Werdnig-Hoffmann's disease. There is prominent psychomotor delay in atonic cerebral palsy, and muscle hypertonia develops in later stages along with the hypotonia. In rickets there are typical changes in vitamin D metabolism, which are not seen in spinal amyotrophy. Oppenheim's myotonia is characterized by relatively preserved motor functions and much more slightly affected respiratory muscles, as well as extremely rare fasciculations. The late form of the disease must be distinguished mainly from Kugelberg-Welander spinal amyotrophy and progressive muscular dystrophies of Duchenne, Erb-Roth, etc.

Treatment. Symptomatic. Drugs stimulating CNS metabolism are used such as Nootropil, Cerebrolysin, Gamalon; as well as agents improving muscle trophy: Methionine, Tocopherol, glutamic acid; products enhancing neuromuscular transmission – Galanthamine, Dibasol, Proserine, anabolic steroids – Retabolil, Dianabol, etc. Kinesitherapy and orthopedic measures preventing joint contractures are also indicated.

I.2. Infantile Chronic Form (Intermediate).

The inheritance of this form of spinal muscular atrophy is autosomal recessive, sporadic.

Pathomorphology. There is loss of anterior horn motoneurons together with atrophy of the anterior roots.

Clinical manifestations. The first symptoms appear as early as the second half of the first year of life. Prominent muscle hypotonia develops, as well as generalized muscle weakness, decreased to absent tendon reflexes, muscle trembling. Pathological changes are more obvious in proximal muscles of the extremities. Sometimes kyphoscoliosis, contractures or other skeleton deformities develop. Psychomotor delay occurs.

The diagnosis is based on the clinical features and laboratory findings which are very similar to those in the severe infantile form. EMG shows increased average duration of potentials and lack of function. Fibrillations are also detected.

The course is slow, progressive. Treatment is symptomatic.

I.3. Juvenile Form or Kugelberg-Welander Disease.
A benign form of spinal muscle atrophy, characterized by slowly progressive muscle
weakness, atrophy and fasciculations predominantly affecting proximal muscles of the extremities.

The incidence is not known.

Etiology and pathogenesis. The disease is inherited in autosomal recessive, autosomal dominant and X-recessive pattern.

Pathomorphology. There are rudimentary and degenerative anterior horn motoneurons, degeneration in the brain stem motor nuclei (IX, X and XII cranial nerves) and demyelinization in the anterior roots. Atrophic changes of muscle fibers and expansion of connective tissue are detected in skeletal muscles.

Clinical manifestations. The disease develops after the age of 4 – 5 years, and sometimes between 14 – 30 years of age. First easy muscle tiredness while moving or running appears. Atrophies develop, initially in proximal muscles of the lower extremities, hip girdle and thighs, gradually affecting the muscles of the arms. Pseudohypertrophy of the calves is almost always observed. The gait is instable, a "duck gait". Scapular winging might develop as a result of shoulder girdle atrophies. Muscle hypotonia in the proximal parts of the limbs occurs. Knee reflexes disappear first; triceps and biceps reflexes disappear later. Fibrillations of the tongue are often seen, but bulbar palsy is very rare. Bone deformities are also infrequent.

Diagnosis and differential diagnosis. The diagnosis is based on genetic studies, clinical features, EMG evidence of neurogenic damage and muscle biopsy. The disorder must be differentiated from progressive muscular dystrophies of Erb-Roth and Becker and Werdnig-Hoffmann spinal muscular atrophy.

The course is slow, progressing for several decades.

I.4. Distal Spinal Muscular Atrophy of Duchenne-Aran.

It is one of the rare forms of spinal muscular atrophy, especially in childhood.

Etiology and pathogenesis. Transmitted in autosomal recessive, autosomal dominant or X-linked recessive pattern. Often sporadic.

Clinical manifestations. The onset of the disease is in the first decade of life. Weakness and gradual atrophy involving the distal muscles of the legs are the first signs. Atrophies in the arms also develop in 25% of patients. This clinical form is characterized by marked foot deformities, early disappearance of ankle reflexes with preserved knee and upper extremity tendon reflexes; no sensory impairment is seen.

Diagnosis and differential diagnosis. The diagnosis is made on the basis of the data from the genealogical analysis, the clinical features and EMG evidence of anterior horn involvement. The condition must be differentiated from Charcot-Marie neural amyotrophy Gowers-Welander distal myopathy.

The course is slow, progressive.

1.5. Spinal Muscular Atrophy in Adults, Vulpian-Bernhard Type.

This is one of the rare forms of spinal amyotrophy, recently regarded by many authors as a subtype of amyotrophic lateral sclerosis.

Etiology and pathogenesis. The disorder is usually considered to be exogenously caused, not genetic. Family transmission is probably about 5 – 10%. A defect in the long arm of chromosome 21 is found in familial cases.

Pathomorphologically there is degeneration in the cells in the anterior horns of the spinal cord.

Clinical manifestations. Pathologic changes: muscle weakness, atrophy and fading of tendon reflexes initially affect the shoulder girdle muscles and the lower limbs later, to the contrary of the other forms of spinal muscular atrophy.

The course is slow, progressive.

Treatment is symptomatic and is not different from that in the other clinical forms of the disorder.

Prophylaxis. Early genetic counseling.

Chapter VII

HEREDITARY POLYNEUROPATHIES

Hereditary neuropathies represent a large heterogenous group of disorders. In some of them impaired functions of the peripheral nerve might be the only presentation of the genetic mutation, whereas in others peripheral neuropathy may be just one of the manifestations of some multisystemic disorder. When classifying hereditary neuropathies it is appropriate to distinguish polyneuropathies with known pathogenesis and metabolic defect and polyneuropathies which pathogenesis is not understood /2, 13, 27/. However it often turns out very difficult to differentiate well between two groups of that kind. Thus when classifying hereditary polyneuropathies one should have in mind a lot of other criteria: the type of inheritance, the age of development, involvement of motor, sensory and/or autonomic structures of peripheral nerves, involvement of other organs and systems, the evolution of the changes, etc. In view of that, hereditary polyneuropathies can be arbitrarily divided into three large groups:
-   I. Hereditary motor and sensory polyneuropathies type I, II, III;
-   II. Hereditary sensory and autonomic polyneuropathies;
-   III. Hereditary polyneuropathies with metabolic disturbance;

1.   Hereditary Motor and Sensory Polyneuropathies Type I, II, III.

1.1. Charcot-Marie-Tooth Disease.

A slow progressive hereditary disease that manifests predominantly with atrophy of distal limb muscles.

Synonyms. Hereditary motor sensory neuropathy /HMSN/ type I, Charcot-Marie-Tooth hypertrophic form of neural muscular atrophy, neural amyotrophy, peroneal atrophy.

Frequency. The incidence of the disease is 1:50 000.

Etiology and pathogenesis. Peroneal muscle atrophy is a syndrome rather than a nosological unit. There are three separate forms according to the clinical manifestations, genealogy and pathology: hypertrophic (demyelinating), neuronal (axonal) and severe form of demyelination, referred to as type I, II and III, respectively.

The inheritance is in autosomal dominant (80%), autosomal recessive (20%) pattern; there are rare sporadic cases /15, 45, 56/.

Pathomorphology. There is degeneration of myelin and axons of the peripheral nerves and roots, as well as anterior horn cell atrophy. Muscle damage is mainly secondary: atrophy, degeneration and disintegration of muscle fibers and connective tissue hyperplasia. The so-called "onion-bulbs" consisting of Schwann cells proliferating around the nerve fibers are pathognomonic /24, 61/.

Clinical manifestations. There are several major forms.

<u>Autosomal Dominant HMSN Type I</u>

The onset is between the first and the second decade of life in most patients /36, 38/. Easy tiredness and weakness while walking or running are the first complaints. They are a consequence of foot or toe deformities. Pes excavatus and hallux flexus develop. The muscles of the shins are hypotonic with marked atrophic changes. The legs resemble inverted bottles - the so-called "stork" legs. A few years later atrophies and pareses also develop in the muscles of the arms. Tendon stretch reflexes are severely reduced, mainly the ankle reflexes. There are sensory disturbances in 2/3 of the patients, with predominant impairment of vibration sense, pain and temperature sensation. Proprioceptic sense is also often affected, and sometimes autonomic sensation as well. Nerve branches become palpably enlarged in some patients. Scoliosis is rare and bulbar paralysis is exceptional /41/.

EMG motor nerve conduction velocity in the upper extremities is between 10 – 35 m/sec.

The course of HMSN type I is of various severity. In general men are more severely affected than women. Symptoms progress slowly, but permanently.

<u>Autosomal Recessive HMSN Type I</u>

The onset is around the age of 10 years. The symptoms are similar to those of the dominant form, but more severe. There is a motor delay. Muscle weakness, atrophy, areflexia and sensory impairment are severe. There is peripheral nerve thickening in a large number of patients which histologically show hypertrophy /57/. EMG demonstrates reduced conduction velocity – about 20 m/sec, which is lower than in the dominant form. The course and symptoms of this form are similar to Friedreich's ataxia, but they show different electrophysiological characteristics and the evolution of the recessive HMSN type I is more favorable /59/.

<u>Autosomal Dominant HMSN Type II</u>

In this form the clinical symptoms develop at a later age. Most patients are in their second decade of life; there are not rare cases of later clinical presentation, up to the age of 60 years.

Pathomorphologically there is axonal degeneration with segmental demyelinization.

Clinical manifestations. The symptoms are similar to those of HMSN type I, but are not so severe. Ataxia and tremor are much less prominent and absence of tendon reflexes is rarer. 50% of the patients do not manifest sensory impairment or bone deformities. The upper limbs are more rarely involved. There is no nerve branch thickening /60/.

Motor conduction velocity in the lower limbs is reduced significantly, whereas in the upper limbs it is normal or in the range of 40 – 50 m/sec.

The course of the disease is slow, progressive and after some time patients stop walking. In this case also men are more severely affected than women. 20 % of the patients are asymptomatic.

Autosomal Recessive HMSN Type II

This form is encountered significantly more rarely and is currently described in a small number of families. The onset is in the age group of 5 to 20 years and the course is more severe in younger patients.

Pathomorphologically there is axonal degeneration and reduction in the density of myelinated fibers is more manifest than in the dominant form.

Clinical manifestations. Progressive muscle weakness and atrophy develop which may affect proximal muscles as well. As time passes until approximately 20 years of age severe pareses develop to a degree when patients are no more able to move. Sensory disturbances and tendon areflexia are often observed while ataxia and scoliosis are rare. There are significant toe deformities and joint contractures in some patients.

Motor conduction velocity varies from 35 m/sec to normal range. EMG is of neurogenic type with fibrillations.

The course is slow and progressive.

Hereditary Motor and Sensory Neuropathy /HMSN/ Type III

This is a rare clinically heterogeneous syndrome transmitted in autosomal recessive pattern. It includes different cases of genetically determined demyelinating polyneuropathies known in the past as Dejerine-Sottas disease.

Etiology and pathogenesis. The type of inheritance is quite various: autosomal dominant, autosomal recessive or sporadic.

Pathomorphology. Pathologically increased transverse diameter of the nerve fibers is seen. "Onion-bulb" formations are observed, consisting of Schwann cells and collagen, along with marked demyelinization /92/.

Clinical manifestations. The onset of the disease is in infancy /63/. Motor development is delayed and is never completed. There is severe muscle hypotonia and muscle atrophies predominantly of the calves and forearms. Later the upper limbs become also involved and muscle contractures develop. There is sensory impairment: pain, paresthesias, tactile and proprioceptive disturbances. Peripheral nerves are palpably enlarged and painful. There are bone deformities too: kyphoscoliosis and synostoses.

The conduction velocity is severely reduced 1 – 10 m/sec; EMG is of neurogenic type. Cerebrospinal fluid protein is elevated.

The course is slow and progressive. Patients become completely disabled no later than 40 – 50 years of age.

2. Hereditary Sensory and Autonomic Neuropathies.

A group of diseases characterized by significant sensory disturbances with concurrent autonomic dysfunctions. They are transmitted in dominant or recessive pattern and sometimes the pattern of inheritance cannot be established.

2.1. Autosomal Dominant Sensory Neuropathy.

The onset is during the second decade of life.

Pathology initially shows damage only to the thin myelinated fibers, but later all myelinated fibers are affected.

Clinical manifestations. An increased threshold for nociception and thermal discrimination occurs in the beginning in the distal parts of the lower limbs, and subsequently other sensory disturbances become apparent. Spontaneous torturing pain in the legs is one of the main characteristics. Mild motor dysfunction may develop. Autonomic symptoms are rare and not typical. A frequent complication in later stages is joint degeneration, most severe in the legs.

The patients' general condition is getting worse slowly but progressively.

2.2. Autosomal Recessive Sensory Neuropathy.

In this form of neuropathy clinical signs appear soon after birth..

Pathomorphological investigation reveals almost complete absence of myelinated fibers and reduced number of nonmyelinated fibers.

Clinically this form of neuropathy is characterized by loss of all sensory modalities, and tactile sensation is more affected than pain and temperature sensation. Sensory disturbances affect distal limb parts and often lead to development of mutilating acropathy, combined with neuropathic joint degeneration, tissue destruction and loss of toes and fingers.

The disease follows a slow progressive course.

2.3. Familial Dysautonomia (Riley-Day Syndrome).

This is a rare condition affecting predominantly Jewish children and characterized by feeding difficulties, vomiting, pulmonary infections and significant autonomic dysfunctions.

Etiology and pathogenesis. Autosomal recessive pattern of inheritance.

Pathomorphology. Neuronal hypoplasia in autonomic ganglia and loss of axons producing catecholamines. There is a significant reduction in the number of nonmyelinated fibers and a lesser one in the number of thin myelinated axons in peripheral nerves.

Clinical manifestations. Severe autonomic disturbances are observed such as decreased lacrimation, poor temperature control, blood pressure variations from postural hypotension to hypertensive crisis, abdominal discomfort and sweat disturbances. The tendon reflexes are absent and pain sensitivity is disturbed. Scoliosis may develop in late stages.

Neurologic symptoms are barely progressive but patients die of recurrent pulmonary infections in early childhood.

2.4. Congenital Sensory Neuropathy with Anhidrosis.

This is a rare disease, transmitted in autosomal recessive pattern, which develops several months after birth.

Pathomorphologically there is selective damage to the thin myelinated fibers and partially to the nonmyelinated axons in Lissauer's zone and in sensory nerves.

Clinical manifestations. There is a motor delay and frequent unexplainable episodes of high fever. Trophic cutaneous lesions and spontaneous bone fracture could be observed along with pain insensitivity and thermal discrimination impairment.

The prognosis of the disorder is unfavorable.

Congenital sensory neuropathy with anhidrosis is also called hereditary sensory and autonomic neuropathy type IV.

2.5. Other Rare Forms of Hereditary Sensory and Autonomic Neuropathies.

Rare conditions of selective loss of thin myelinated fibers and preserved nonmyelinated fibers and thick myelinated fibers are described.

The clinical course is characterized by selective loss of pain sensation that may affect the distal parts of the limbs only or may be diffuse. There is also sweat disturbance.

These patients are classified into hereditary sensory and autonomic neuropathy type V.

3. Hereditary Neuropathies with Metabolic Disturbance.

This is a large group of neuropathies with a known metabolic defect which is genetically transmitted. It includes hereditary amyloidoses, porphyries, lipidoses and conditions associated with impaired deoxyribonucleic acid /DNA/ repair.

3.1. Hereditary Amyloidoses.

There are four types of hereditary neuropathies caused by intracellular deposition of amyloid.

Etiology and pathogenesis. All forms of amyloid neuropathy are inherited in autosomal dominant pattern. Deposition of amyloid in peripheral nerves, sensory and autonomic ganglia is considered to play a major role in the pathogenesis.

3.1.1. Type I (ANDRADE).

This is the most common form of amyloid polyneuropathy. The onset of the disease is between 30 – 40 years and rarely later.

Pathomorphologically there is deposition of amyloid in the vitreous body, renal parenchyma and the heart as well as in peripheral nerves. Nerve biopsy shows amyloid deposition in the endoneural space and in perineural blood vessels. Myelinated fibers are well preserved, whereas nonmyelinated fibers are significantly reduced. Electron microscopy shows typical non-branching amyloid fibrils 7- 10 nm in width. The amyloid of these fibers does not contain the amino acids cysteine or tryptophan.

Clinical manifestations. There is gradual fading of pain and thermal sensation in the lower limbs together with pain and paresthesias. With time sensory disturbances involve the upper limbs too. In terminal stages of the disease the vibratory and proprioceptive sense is loss, distal muscle atrophy and tendon areflexia develop. Autonomic dysfunctions are manifested as postural hypotension, anhidrosis, impotency, bladder dysfunction and visual disturbances. Neurogenic arthropathies and trophic skin ulcerations may develop.

The condition progresses slowly and patients die in about 10 years after the onset of the disease due to infections and renal failure.

3.1.2 Type II (RUKAVINA).

This form develops in patients over 40 years of age and follows a more favorable course than the first one.

Pathomorphologically there is marked amyloid infiltration of the blood vessels of many organs, the peripheral nerves and the vitreous body.

Clinical manifestations. Bilateral symmetric syndrome of median nerve compression and carpal tunnel syndrome is observed. Gradually generalized sensory and autonomic polyneuropathy develops, more prevalent in the lower limbs.

The condition follows a slowly progressive course.

3.1.3 Type III (VAN-ALLEN).

The clinical features of this form are very similar to those of type I, but autonomic dysfunctions are much more severe. There is high incidence of duodenal ulcer in these patients.

3.1.4 Type IV (MERETOJA).

The onset is at approximately 30 years of age with visual deficit caused by corneal lusterless. There are cranial nerve lesions, dystrophic changes in the cornea and poor skin turgor along with the manifestations of neuropathy /18/.

3.2. Hereditary Neuropathies in Acute Intermittent Porphyria, Cutaneous Hepatic Porphyria and Hereditary Coproporpyiria.

Frequency. 1:13 000 to 1: 18 000 in some countries. Women are affected more often than men. Cutaneous hepatic porphyria and hereditary coproporphyria are relatively less frequent. The usual age of presentation is 20 – 40.

Etiology and pathogenesis. All three forms of hereditary porphyric neuropathy are transmitted in autosomal dominant pattern. Synthesis of heme is affected in porphyrias. In acute intermittent porphyria there is deficit of uroporphyrinogen I synthetase which blocks the metabolic pathway of heme synthesis and accumulation of delta-aminolevulinic acid and porphobilinogen. During periods of disease aggravation the excessive amounts of these neurotoxic substances are excreted in urine. The pathogenesis of cutaneous hepatic porphyria is similar. Hereditary coproporphyria is caused by deficiency of the enzyme coproporphyrin oxydase /28/.

Pathomorphology. There is axonal degeneration of nerve radicles innervating proximal muscle groups and loss of anterior horn cells.

Clinical manifestations. The disorder is characterized by crises of crampy abdominal pain and polyneuropathies. The abdominal colics are accompanied by nausea, vomiting, constipation. Autonomic dysfunction is also frequent, including tachycardia, hyperthermia, oliguria, etc. In some severe cases cardiac, renal or hepatic failure or paralytic ileus may develop which are life-threatening conditions. Epileptic seizures and psychoses are seen more rarely. After these symptoms fade away, a polyneuropathy develops, including flaccid paralyses in proximal muscles of the lower limbs and later involving the upper limbs as well. There is a pronounced pain syndrome and other sensory disturbances. The early appearance of muscle atrophies is characteristic of this type of polyneuropathy. In some cases the caudal group of the cranial nerves might be affected with development of respiratory complications.

Diagnosis. The diagnostic tests of Noesch and Swartz-Watson are used; they detect qualitatively porphobilinogen in urine /58, 86/.

The course of the disease is slow, progressive. Crises are sometimes provoked by intercurrent infections or some drugs (barbiturates). Death occurs with involvement of respiratory muscles.

3.3. Hereditary Polyneuropathies Caused by Disturbances in Lipid Metabolism.

3.3.1. Hereditary Polyneuropathy in HDL-deficiency.
Synonyms. Tangier disease.

Etiology and pathogenesis. Transmitted in autosomal recessive pattern. In patients' plasma the level of high density α-lipoproteins is significantly lowered. Plasma cholesterol is also decreased; whereas the level of triglycerides is normal or even increased. Complex cholesterol esters are deposited in different tissues such as bone marrow, spleen, skin, etc. Peripheral nerves are involved in many patients /83/.

Pathomorphology. There is degeneration of nonmyelinated and thin myelinated fibers and accumulation of neutral fats and complex cholesterol esters in Schwann cells.

Clinical manifestations. The onset is either during childhood, or during adulthood. There are two variants of the disease course. In the first one symptoms of mononeuropathy predominate. In the second one generalized polyneuropathy develops together with muscle weakness of the palms and face, tendon areflexia and nociceptive and thermal discrimination impairment. These disturbances may resemble sensory dissociation of syringomyelic type.

The course is slow, progressive.

3.4. Adrenoleukodystrophy and Adrenomyeloneuropathy.
Adrenoleukodystrophy is a X-linked recessive disorder. The exact metabolic defect has not been established, but increased ratio of C-26 and C-22 fatty acids in skin fibroblasts is found in patients and carriers.

Clinical manifestations of the disease include progressive dementia, epileptic seizures, quadripareses, amaurosis and adrenal insufficiency. Adrenomyeloneuropathy develops concurrently.

It is characterized clinically by distal muscle weakness, sensory impairment and spastic paraplegia.

Progression is slow and permanent /62/.

3.5. Cockayne Syndrome.

The syndrome includes a delay in physical development, mental retardation, pigmentary retinopathy and increased photosensitivity. Moreover, symptoms of polyneuropathy are seen: hyporeflexia, low conduction velocity in peripheral nerves, loss of myelinated fibers and segmental nerve demyelinization /48/.

Hereditary polyneuropathies caused by disturbances in lipid metabolism are also observed in metachromatic leukodystrophy, Krabbe disease, abetalipoproteinemia or Bassen-Kornzweig syndrome, Refsum disease, Fabry disease, etc. /described in chapter III and IV/.

3.6. Hereditary Polyneuropathies Associated with Disturbed DNA-repair.

3.6.1 Xeroderma Pigmentosum.

It begins as a dermatologic condition and is characterized by increased sensitivity to ultraviolet light.

Etiology and pathogenesis. The disease is transmitted in autosomal recessive pattern. Genetically there are six subgroups.

Pathomorphology. Severe loss of thick myelinated fibers in peripheral nerves is found. Biochemical investigations show defective DNA-repair.

Clinical manifestations. The onset is manifested by reduced to absent tendon and periostal reflexes, and later pain, paresthesias, etc. develop. Nerve conduction investigation demonstrates changes in the action potentials of sensory nerves. Other neurologic symptoms present also: microcephaly and mental retardation, epileptic seizures, spasticity and cerebellar ataxia.

4. Diagnosis and Differential Diagnosis of Hereditary Polyneuropathies.

The diagnosis is based on the genealogical analysis showing the pattern of inheritance (autosomal recessive, autosomal dominant or X-linked) and the history for onset of symptoms in childhood or adulthood. Secondly the diagnosis is established based on the knowledge of the features of the clinical course (distal limb atrophies, polyneuropathic sensory impairment, slow symptom progression). EMG shows low conduction velocity in peripheral nerves, and biopsy demonstrates the pathomorphological changes /11, 49/. Sporadic cases are particularly difficult to diagnose. Then it is important to find out the specific features of each polyneuropathy, for example teleangiectasias in Louis-Bar syndrome.

Differential diagnosis is made in two directions. First, separate forms of hereditary neuropathies must be distinguished from each other, and secondly, hereditary neuropathies must be distinguished from secondary neuropathies. Thus, in sporadic cases of amyloid polyneuropathies the hereditary pathogenesis can be confirmed only if another family member becomes sick with the same disease. The onset of hereditary polyneuropathies in childhood or adulthood is also of great importance in clinical diagnostics. Most neuropathies beginning in childhood, which present in multisystemic disorders, are hereditary in nature. Thus if neuropathy is accompanied by ataxia, Louis-Bar syndrome, Friedreich's disease, xeroderma pigmentosum, HMSN type I, etc. should be suspected. In case of coexistence of neuropathy and mental retardation, metachromatic leukodystrophy, Fabry disease, etc. must be set on mind. Distinguishing motor from motor sensory neuropathies presents significant difficulties. When demyelinating neuropathy occurs with markedly decreased conduction velocity, differential diagnosis is made between Refsum disease, HMSN type I and type III and idiopathic inflammatory neuropathy. Precise clinical and EMG investigation of parents and siblings are needed for their differentiation, because HMSN type I can be transmitted by asymptomatic family members, particularly females.

Some hereditary neuropathies in adults share the characteristic features of Refsum disease, Fabry disease and Tangier disease. In contrast to them HMSN type I, II and III show no specific symptoms. Slowly progressive, predominantly axonal, motor neuropathies present a diagnostic problem in adults. They are distinguished from HMSN type II mainly by genetic investigation.

Hereditary polyneuropathies must be differentiated from secondary polyneuropathies such as hereditary distal spinal amyotrophy, myotonic dystrophy, distal myopathies and infectious and toxic polyneuritis, etc.

5. Treatment of Hereditary Polyneuropathies.

Therapy aims at improving muscle trophics and nerve conduction. For this purpose drugs based on adenosine triphosphoric acid , cocarboxylase, leucine and glutamic acid, etc. are given. Vitamins E, A, B and C are largely used. Vitamin E is highly effective, particularly in abetalipoproteinemias at a dose of 100 mg/kg/24h. Medications improving microcirculation are indicated – Pentoxyphylline, Nicotinic acid, etc. Anticholinesterase agents such as Proserine, Galanthamine and Oxazyl improve neuromuscular conduction. A dietary and hygienic regimen is also effective in certain conditions. Thus in Refsum disease restriction of foods containing phytanic acid is beneficial; and in porphyrias it is necessary to avoid drugs like barbiturates, Tegretol, Methyldopa, oral contraceptives, etc. Physiotherapy and kinesitherapy are also largely applied for maintaining patients motor activity. In some cases orthopedic procedures are also needed to correct the deformities.

Treatment should be individually based, complex and continuous.

6. Genetic Counseling in Hereditary Polyneuropathies.

Genetic counseling in hereditary polyneuropathies is a quite pressing issue because there is no effective treatment available. The risk of occurrence of the disease in the newborns in autosomal dominant pattern of transmission is 50 %. This is the case in amyloid neuropathy, porphyrias and dominant forms of HMSN. Problems occur when it is not possible to determine the carrier of the pathologic gene before their children are born, which is the case in amyloid neuropathy ANDRADE type. Heterozygotes in acute intermittent porphyria can be identified by low activity of the enzyme uroporphyrinogen I synthetase. In this case the findings are similar in the carriers of the gene and the healthy individuals from control groups. No more than 10% of cases with predominant autosomal dominant pattern of inheritance follow a severe clinical course. When counseling children of siblings whose parents have suffered from HMSN type I, a low conduction velocity in peripheral nerves is found from early childhood independent of the absence or presence of clinical manifestations. Thus, healthy people without clinical or electrophysiological abnormalities are at low risk for having sick children. It is more complicated in cases of autosomal recessive inheritance. If the disease is present in more than one sibling of healthy parents, the risk for occurrence of HMSN in this generation of the patient is 1:4. The risk is much higher in marriages between cousins. In Refsum disease, Krabbe disease, metachromatic leukodystrophy, Louis-Bar syndrome, abetalipoproteinemia and Riley-Day syndrome the inheritance is in autosomal recessive pattern, i.e. the risk is 25%. Other conditions such as Fabry disease, adrenomyeloneuropathy and adrenoleukodystrophy are inherited in X-linked recessive pattern, i.e. half of the sons of female carriers develop clinical manifestations, and half of their daughters are also carriers. Sons of affected males remain healthy, but all daughters of affected males are carriers of the pathologic gene.

The main purpose of genetic counseling is to explain the risk of hereditary polyneuropathy and to prevent transmission of the disease.

Chapter VIII

HEREDITARY MYOPATHIES

A group of diseases characterized by primary dystrophic changes in muscle tissue. Myopathies are transmitted in different patterns (autosomal dominant, autosomal recessive and X-linked recessive), different muscle groups are involved, and their course is chronic and progressive. The common clinical manifestations include development of flaccid paralyses, together with decreased or absent tendon and periostal reflexes, slowly progressive, symmetric muscular atrophies, EMG demonstrating voluntary action potentials of shorter duration and lowered amplitude, with no evidence of neurogenic lesion. Biochemical tests show increased level of serum creatine kinase (CK) and aldolase, elevated creatine and decreased level of creatinine in urine as a result of enhanced muscle disintegration /29, 77/.

I. Progressive Muscular Dystrophies (PMD).

A heterogenous group of hereditary diseases of skeletal muscles characterized by a slow and progressive course.

Pathogenesisof PMD is unclear. They probably develop in cases of certain structural or functional defects in the plasma membrane of myofibers. This could explain the efflux of glycogen, myoglobin, potassium and other substances from the sarcoplasm to the extracellular matrix and the blood stream and the increased activity of some enzymes in plasma, such as creatine kinase. Recent researches show that disturbed calcium metabolism in muscle fibers plays an important role for the development of the dystrophic process in skeletal muscles – increased calcium influx in mitochondria leads to their damage. Elevated calcium concentration in muscle fibers causes their hypercontraction and tearing.

Pathomorphological changes depend directly on the stage of the clinical evolution. Initially the myofibril size is changed with small areas of degeneration and proliferation of connective tissue. As the condition progresses darkening of the fibers, increased calcium concentration and myofibril tearing are observed. In late stages degeneration is significant and almost all muscle tissue is replaced by connective and adipose tissue. There is proliferation of vascular adventitia, narrowing of the vascular lumen and sometimes perimural thrombi. Histochemically, increased level of acid mucopolysaccharides in muscle and collagen fibers is found.

PMD are a heterogenous group of diseases. Differences among separate forms include the pattern of inheritance, the age of onset, the muscle groups affected and the progression of atrophies. On the basis of these PMD are divided into the following types:

1. X-linked recessive forms:
    a) Duchenne progressive muscular dystrophy;
    b) Becker-Kiener progressive muscular dystrophy;
    c) Dreifuss progressive muscular dystrophy;
2. Girdle forms /"limb-girdle" forms/:
    a) Infantile form;
    b) Juvenile form: Erb-Rott type;
    c) Adult form;
3. Facioscapulohumeral form.
4. Scapuloperoneal form.
5. Congenital forms:
    a) Malignant type;
    b) Benign type;
6. Distal form: Welander type.
7. Ophthalmic and oculopharyngeal form and other rare forms.

1.1. Duchenne Progressive Muscular Dystrophy.

Frequency. The incidence of the disease is 3.3:100 000 of the population and 14:100 000 of newborns.

Etiology and pathogenesis. The disorder is transmitted in X-linked recessive pattern. Mostly boys suffer from this condition. Girls are rarely affected although this is possible in cases of karyotype X0, mosaicism X0/XX, X0/XXX, X0/XXX/XX and structural chromosome abnormalities.

Pathomorphology. Marked degenerative changes in muscle fibers with areas of necrosis, phagocytosis and expansion of connective and adipose tissue in place of myofibrils are seen. _

Clinical manifestations. The onset is between the age of 1 and 3 years. There is an apparent motor delay: children experience difficulties in sitting, standing and walking. Their movements are clumsy, often stagger, stumble and fall. Muscle tiredness, general weakness, especially with prolonged walking and climbing stairs, develop around the age of 2. Compensatory lumbar hyperlordosis is seen because of hip girdle and axial muscle weakness. The typical "duck" gait is observed. The child uses the hands to climb up the legs in order to assume an upright position /Gowers sign/, which is characteristic. Muscular atrophies are always symmetrical. In the beginning they involve proximal muscles of the lower limbs, the hip girdle and the thighs but later follow an ascending course to muscles of the upper limbs, the shoulder girdle and the back. Lordosis, loose joints, scapular winging and a wasp waist appear because of the atrophies. Pseudohypertrophy of the calves is a classic feature. Facial muscle weakness is a late event: the so-called "tapir face appearance". In the terminal stages all muscle groups are affected and respiratory failure develops. Neurologic examination determines hypotonia predominantly in proximal muscles. Tendon stretch reflexes change in certain order. In early stages of the disease knee reflexes disappear, followed by disappearance of biceps and triceps reflexes, and ankle reflexes fade last. There are no sensory or pyramidal disturbances. Cardiovascular, skeletal and endocrine involvement is typical of this type of PMD. Bone and joint damage include deformities of the spinal column, thorax and feet. Roentgenograms show narrowed cortical layer of long bones and diaphyses. Cardiovascular involvement is clinically manifested by blood pressure and heart rate variations, and more rarely by heart failure and rhythm disturbances. Myocardial damage cause

ECG changes: abnormal R/S ratio in V1 and abnormal Q in V6. Neuroendocrine disturbances are encountered in about half of the patients. Adiposogenital dystrophy and Cushing's syndrome are most common. Intellectual decline varies from mild to profound mental retardation but it is not parallel to motor changes.

Diagnosis and differential diagnosis. The diagnosis is based on the evidence from genetic investigation concerning the transmission pattern (X-linked recessive), the clinical features (early appearance of symmetrical muscular atrophies of proximal muscle groups of the lower limbs which ascend, severe cardiac and endocrine disturbances). A pathognomonic laboratory finding is the highly elevated level of creatine kinase even in early stages of the disease. Creatinuria is also common. EMG shows decreased amplitudes, oscillations and polyphasic potentials. Muscle biopsy confirms the diagnosis /67/. The disease must be distinguished from Werdnig-Hoffmann spinal muscular atrophy, rickets and other forms of PMD.

Evolution. Rapid and malignant progression. At the age of about 7 – 10 years all motor functions are severely affected; patients become completely handicapped at the age of about 14 – 15 years and die of respiratory complications and infections.

1.2. Becker-Kiener Progressive Muscular Dystrophy.
The incidence of this form is not known.

Etiology and pathogenesis. X-linked recessive pattern of inheritance. Recent evidence from gene mapping via DNA restriction enzymes indicate that the mutations, similar to Duchenne PMD, are localized in the short arm of X-chromosome – Xp21 - and are allelic (different mutations in the same gene locus). Different from Duchenne PMD where the amount of dystrophin (an important component of myofibrils) is extremely low, in Becker dystrophy this protein is produced in sufficient quality, but its molecular structure is changed /37/.

Clinical manifestations. The firsts symptoms appear around the age of 10- 15 years. General muscle weakness develops, as well as pathologic muscle tiredness at physical strain and pseudohypertrophy of the calves. Muscular atrophies are symmetrical and initially affect proximal muscle groups of the lower limbs, and later ascend. A "duck" gait and difficulties in assuming an upright position occur. A milder hypotonia than in Duchenne PMD is evident. Tendon reflexes are affected more rarely, except knee reflexes which fade early. Cardiovascular disturbances are also less prominent. Endocrine problems usually include gynecomastia and impotence. Patients' intellect is preserved.

Diagnosis and differential diagnosis. The diagnosis is suggested by the genealogic analysis, the clinical manifestations (late onset around 10 – 15 years of age with development of proximal muscle atrophies), biochemical changes (elevated plasma creatine phosphokinase and lactate dehydrogenase), EMG and morphological changes. The disease must be distinguished from Duchenne PMD, Kugelberg-Welander spinal muscular atrophy, etc.

Evolution. The course is more favorable. Patients remain ambulatory until the age of 40 or later.

1.3. Dreifuss Progressive Muscular Dystrophy.

The incidence of this form is not known. It is transmitted in X-linked recessive pattern. The main characteristic is the strikingly rapid expansion of connective tissue in muscles.

Clinical manifestations. The onset is at the age of 5 – 7 years. As in the other forms of PMD, progressive muscle weakness and pathologic muscle tiredness during motion and physical strain occur. Muscular atrophies affect symmetric parts of the muscles of the lower limbs, hip girdle and thighs. Proximal muscle groups of the legs are involved much later. A distinctive feature of this type of muscular dystrophy is the early development of elbow contractures and retraction of the Achilles tendons. The dystrophic process affects the heart as well with development of rhythm disturbances. Patients' intellect is preserved.

Diagnosis and differential diagnosis. The diagnosis is based on the pattern of inheritance and the clinical features (onset in early childhood with slowly progressive atrophies, beginning in the legs and early development of elbow contractures). EMG, morphological changes showing primary dystrophic alterations in skeletal muscles, as well as the elevated serum creatine phosphokinase /CPK/ are also important. The disease must be distinguished from other forms of primary muscular dystrophies and spinal muscular atrophy, as well as from myositis, polyarthritis and deforming spondylosis.

Evolution. The course is slowly progressive.

1.4 Girdle Forms ("Limb-Girdle" Forms).

This group is heterogenous, including many different types according to the age of onset and the muscles damaged. Patients are in the age group between 1 and 50 years of age. Sometimes the primary muscular involvement begins from the hip girdle muscles, and other times the shoulder girdle is affected first. The juvenile form of Erb-Rott is the most common condition from this group of dystrophies.

1.4.1 Progressive Muscular Dystrophy Erb-Rott Type.

Frequency. 1.5:100 000 of the population.

It is inherited in autosomal recessive pattern. The defective gene is localized in the long arm of chromosome 15. Sporadic forms are common. Males and females are equally affected.

Pathomorphology shows primary muscular damage which is typical for PMD.

Clinical manifestations. The first signs of the disorder appear around the age of 14 – 16 years, rarely earlier. Muscle weakness and increased physical tiredness occur. Atrophies initially affect proximal muscle groups of the lower limbs. Sometimes muscles of the hip and the shoulder girdle are affected by the dystrophic process at the same time. There are difficulties in climbing stairs and assuming an upright position. Later axial and upper limb muscles become involved. Because of the atrophies lordosis, scapular winging and wasp waist develop. In attempt to lift up the patient suspending them under the arms, the shoulders rise up easily and the head hangs down between them – "the symptom of free shoulders". A "duck" gait appears; the face is hypomimic - "sphynx face" with "tapir lips". Muscle pseudohypertrophy, joint contractures and tendon retraction are moderate. Tendon reflexes, mainly the knee and the biceps and triceps reflexes, weaken and disappear early. Gradually the diffuse damage to muscle tissue involves smooth muscles of internal organs, as well as cardiac muscles. The peristalsis becomes weak; respiratory or heart failure might develop.

Diagnosis and differential diagnosis. The diagnosis is based on the data from the genetic investigation, the clinical manifestations (onset at the age of about 14 – 15, localization of the atrophies, rapid progression of symptoms), EMG and muscle biopsy. The condition must be distinguished from the other forms of PMD and from Kugelberg-Welander spinal muscular atrophy.

Evolution. Rapidly progressing. Patient very soon become completely handicapped.

1.5. Facioscapulohumeral Muscular Dystrophy (Landouzi-Dejerine Disease).

Frequency. 0.9 to 2:100 000 of the population. Transmitted in autosomal dominant pattern. The gene defect is localized in the long arm of chromosome 4. Males and females are equally affected.

Clinical manifestations. The onset is between 10 and 20 years of life. Muscle weakness and atrophies are localized in facial mimic muscles, shoulder girdle muscles and biceps and triceps brachii muscles. Because of the atrophy the face becomes hypomimic. The absence of wrinkles on the forehead, the "transverse smile" and the "tapir lips" are typical. Brachial and shoulder muscle atrophies determine the appearance of "free shoulder" symptom, scapular winging and scoliosis. Atrophy often involves lower limb muscles as well. Then prominent pseudohypertrophy of the calves is observed. Muscle tone is decreased first in proximal muscles of the lower limbs. Tendon reflexes are decreased, predominantly in the arms /32/.

Diagnosis and the differential diagnosis are similar to the other forms of PMD.

Evolution. It is slow. Patients preserve their work capacity for a long period of time.

1.6. Scapuloperoneal Muscular Dystrophy.

This disorder has a relatively late onset: between 25 and 30 years of age. It is considered to be an intermediate form between primary myopathies and neural muscular atrophy. It is inherited in autosomal dominant pattern. Distal muscle groups of the lower limbs and proximal muscle groups of the upper limbs are affected by degeneration. Besides atrophies, coarse fasciculations and early disappearance of tendon reflexes might be observed. Mild sensory impairment may be detected in a number of cases as distal hypesthesia, paresthesia or pain.

EMG shows specific for this form changes – dysrhythmic oscillations at rest, low amplitude and sometimes grouped spikes in active movement /20/.

1.7. Congenital Muscular Dystrophies.

This group includes some very rare forms of hereditary progressive muscular dystrophies with malignant or benign clinical course.

1.7.1. Nemaline Rod Myopathy.

It is inherited in autosomal dominant pattern, but sporadic forms are not rare.

Pathomorphologically there is accumulation of specific bodies, exceeding the length of myofibrils, in muscles, predominantly in type I fibers. They are colored in red when Gomori trichrome stain is used. Ultrastructurally, they are fibrillar elements originating from the Z-band of muscle cells. Nemaline structures are found in almost all muscle fibers. There are no changes in the rest of the muscle tissue.

Clinical manifestations. The symptoms may be observed at birth or during the first year of life. Slowly progressive or steady muscle weakness and limb hypotrophy develop, together with absence of tendon reflexes. Cranial muscles are also affected. There are skeletal deformities too: protruding facial part of the skull, thoracic, feet and spinal column deformities, sometimes arachnodactyly. So children look like patients with Marfan's syndrome. Proximal muscle groups are most severely affected.

EMG presents evidence of primary muscle damage. Serum CPK is insignificantly elevated.

Evolution. Most cases of the disease are benign and nonprogressive. There are single cases of malignant evolution reported.

1.7.2. Central Core Myopathy.

Synonyms. Central core disease, Shy and Magee disease.

This disorder is named after the typical morphological changes: an abnormal bundle of myofibrils is formed in the center of almost each muscle fiber.

The transmission is autosomal dominant with reduced penetrance.

Pathomorphologically there is complete absence of fibers type II.

A homogenous central zone colored in blue and a peripheral pink zone is seen in fibers type I if Gomori trichrome stain is used. Under the electron microscope, almost complete absence of mitochondria and reduction of the elements of the sarcotubular system and glycogen is evident in the central areas of muscle fibers as well. Fibrillar space is extremely narrowed and configuration of the Z-zone is altered.

Clinical manifestations. Muscle hypotonia and weakness predominantly affecting proximal muscle groups is evident from the first days of life. The lower limbs are more severely affected than the arms. Muscle hypotonia is mild, and tendon reflexes are preserved. Children learn to walk later, but nevertheless develop normal motor skills. There are also bone and joint deformities: equinovarus deformities, kyphoscoliosis, etc. Patients' intellect is normal.

Evolution. The course is slow and relatively nonprogressive.

1.7.3. Myotubular Myopathy.

Synonyms. Centronuclear myopathy.

This form is inherited in autosomal recessive pattern. Pathomorphologically muscle fibers are of seriously reduced size with a central nucleus, reminding of the structure of embryonic muscle tissue. This gives the name of this form of PMD. Under the electron microscope there are areas of degeneration in myofibrils and increased activity of mitochondrial enzymes is proven histochemically.

Clinical manifestations. The disorder presents at birth or in early childhood. Progressive weakness in proximal muscles, and sometimes distal muscles as, is observed. Later atrophies of axial, mimic, ocular and respiratory muscles develop. Bone deformities might be observed, predominantly scoliosis. EMG demonstrates coexistence of myopathic changes and spontaneous activity.

Evolution. The disorder progresses rapidly. Heterozygotic carriers of the pathologic gene have subclinical damage to muscle tissue with milder involvement of muscle fibers.

1.8. Mitochondrial Myopathies.

Different forms of myopathies in childhood have been described, in which the earliest and most prominent changes are those of mitochondria /68/.

1.8.1. Megaconial Myopathy.

Synonyms. Shy and Gonatal disease.

It is inherited in autososmal recessive pattern. Giant mitochondria (1 – 2 micrometers in diameter) are found histochemically and by electron microscopy in patients' muscles, especially in muscle fibers type I. Moreover there is intracellular accumulation of fat histochemically.

Clinically the disease is characterized by rapid progression of severe muscular atrophies, early disappearance of tendon reflexes and severe skeletal deformities. Patients become completely disabled in a few months or years.

1.8.2. Megaconial Myopathy with Hypermetabolism.

It is inherited in autosomal recessive pattern. Pathomorphologically there is moderately pronounced degeneration in muscle tissue. Electron microscopy demonstrates a large amount of mitochondria of various sizes, containing folded or oval structures and altered internal architectonic. The quantity of total mitochondrial protein is increased and so is the cytochrome oxydase activity, in some mitochondria hypermetabolism is evident as a result of phosphate acceptor impairment and the increased activity of endogenous ATP.

Clinical manifestations. Children have high fever, profuse sweating, polyphagia and, tachycardia and weight loss. A severe syndrome of myopathy including muscle atrophies, absence of tendon reflexes, creatinuria and characteristic myopathic EMG findings develops. The level of basic metabolism is significantly increased and ranges from 140% to 210%. Respiratory complications might occur.

1.8.3. Pleoconial Myopathy.

Synonyms. Shy's disease.

This form of PMD is also transmitted in autosomal recessive pattern. Massive proliferation of mitochondria, enlarged several times, that damage fibrillar architectonic of muscle tissue is found pathomorphologically. There are also fibers with central nuclei and moderate expansion of connective tissue.

Clinical manifestations include flaccid movements from birth, delayed physical development and muscle weakness. Periodically attacks of profuse sweating, thirst, nausea and vomiting occur.

The course is progressive, although not very rapid.

1.8.4. Congenital Malignant Muscular Dystrophy.

Autosomal recessive transmission. Pathomorphologic investigation shows severe atrophy and loss of muscle fibers of the body and extremities and expansion of connective tissue. The nuclei are localized in the center of the myofibrils. No signs of regeneration in muscle tissue are noted.

Clinically this nosological form is characterized by eyelid ptosis, swallowing disturbances and early development of severe joint contractures. Children die of severe respiratory complications during the first year of life.

1.8.5. Distal Myopathy.

It is extremely rare. The transmission is in autosomal dominant pattern with reduced penetrance. Males are affected more often.

Degeneration in limb distal muscle groups is evident pathologically.

Clinical manifestations. The disorder begins at a later age: between 20 and 25 years. Initially muscular atrophies involve the knees, feet, palms and arms and later other muscle groups become affected. Tendon stretch reflexes disappear early, there are no fasciculations or sensory impairment. EMG shows normal motor and sensory conduction velocity. The clinical course is slowly progressive.

1.8.6. Ocular and Oculopharyngeal Myopathy.
A rare form of myopathy which is transmitted in autosomal dominant pattern with very low penetrance. Sporadic forms are more common.

Degeneration in external ocular muscles and pharyngeal muscles is seen pathologically.

Clinical features present in adulthood, but onset during puberty is also possible. External ocular muscles are affected selectively which is manifested clinically by ptosis without diplopia. The orbicular ocular muscles and forehead muscles are frequently involved. When pharyngeal and laryngeal muscles are affected, we speak of oculopharyngeal myopathy. Sometimes cervical and shoulder girdle muscles are involved, though less severely.

The diagnosis is based on the genetic investigation and the clinical manifestations. The disease should be distinguished from ocular myasthenia, basal tumors or inflammation and mesencephalic tumors.

The course is slowly progressive.

1.9. Treatment of PMD.
There is no etiologic treatment available. Symptomatic medications are applied in 2 or 3 courses a year. Vitamins B, C and E, ATP, Nootropil, Encephabol, Cerebrolysin, etc. are used /53, 79, 90/. Good, though short-lived, effect is observed with anticholinesterase agents: Mestinon, Proserine and Galanthamine. Physiotherapy and kinesitherapy also play an important role in therapy. Orthopedic procedures are often performed: elongation of the tendon of m. triceps sure, removing forward the tendons of feet flexors, surgical correction of scoliosis, splint placement, etc. Respiratory gymnastics

has a prophylactic effect, as well as early antibiotic treatment of upper respiratory tract infections, etc. /87/.

1.10. Genetic Counseling.

Estimating the risk of transmission in autosomal dominant and autosomal recessive pattern (50% and 25%, respectively) is not very difficult. Obscurity occurs in Duchenne and Becker muscular dystrophies because of transmission of the disease from clinically healthy carriers to half of their sons. Another milestone is represented by the issue whether a single case of Duchenne PMD is a new mutation (there is no risk of transmission from female relatives) or the mother is a carrier and there are no other sick males in the family. Finding the carriers and prenatal diagnosis is possible only if DNA analysis is applied. DNA probes and restriction enzymes are used and polymorphism in certain fragments of the DNA sequence is proven. These fragments are bound to the locus or include portions of the pathologic gene itself. Therefore all family members of a patient with PMD must be tested.

2. Metabolic Myopathies.

This group consists of several congenital myopathies which develop when certain defects in electrolyte, glycogen or lipid metabolism, etc. are present.

2.1. Periodic Paralyses.

A group of rare genetic conditions characterized by defective potassium metabolism, resulting in decreased muscle excitability.

Synonyms. Paroxysmal myoplegia, paroxysmal paralysis, familial paroxysmal paralysis, Westphal's disease, Cavaré-Westphal syndrome, Cavaré-Romberg syndrome, Laverie syndrome, Cavaré-Westphal periodic limb palsy.

Etiology and pathogenesis. It is transmitted in autosomal dominant pattern with a strong penetrance. Predominantly boys are affected.

Pathomorphologically there is a great number of vacuoles in muscle tissue, as well as connective tissue expansion. Electron microscopy shows widening of cisterns and sarcoplasmic reticulum.

There are no pathologic changes in the central or peripheral nervous system.

Clinical manifestations. There are 3 basic forms of periodic paralyses: hypokalemic, hyperkalemic and normokalemic.

2.1.1. Hypokalemic Periodic Paralysis.

The onset is usually in childhood, more rarely in adolescence. It is believed that in this form the sodium pump in myofibrils is not effective, and therefore increased sodium influx results and hypokalemia develops.

The disease is characterized by periodically repetitive episodes of sudden muscle weakness which sometimes causes plegia of the body and limbs. In general, cervical and facial muscles are not affected, although there are cases of mimic, pharyngeal and respiratory muscle weakness. There are reports of death during the episode of paralysis. Muscle weakness is most prominent in proximal limb muscles. Complete atonia and tendon areflexia are present. Significant autonomic dysfunction often develops: hyperhidrosis, hyperemia of the face and the upper part of the body, shortness of breath and arrhythmias. The attacks of muscle weakness usually occur at night or early in the morning and are sometimes preceded by mild muscle weakness. Most such episodes last a few hours. They fade away sooner if the patient is moving, whereas rest provokes them and makes them more intense. Other precipitating factors include emotional stress, cold exposure and alcohol consumption. Between the episodes, the muscle strength, tone and reflexes are usually preserved.

During an attack the serum level of potassium is severely decreased and reaches 1.4 – 1.6 mmol/l. The level of phosphorus is decreased too, whereas the sodium level and glucose concentration are increased. Complete bioelectrical silence is registered on EMG. ECG shows negative T-wave in leads II and III.

2.1.2. Hyperkalemic Periodic Paralysis.

Synonyms. Ganstorp syndrome, hyperkalemic myoplegia, hereditary episodic adynamia, adynamia-hyperkalemia.

It develops at an earlier age than the hypokalemic form. Hyperkalemic periodic paralysis is considered to be a result of potassium pump defect which leads to abnormal potassium reabsorption. This is the cause for accumulation of potassium /31/.

Different from the hypokalemic form, in this case the episodes of muscle weakness occur during daytime and are of considerably shorter duration. The attacks are provoked by intensive physical strain and underfeeding and fade away quickly following glucose intake. Muscle weakness is most prominent in distal muscle groups and in cranial muscles. Facial and limb paresthesias are common. Tendon reflexes are preserved or even increased. During an attacks hyperkalemia and hypoglycemia are detected in patients' sera.

2.1.3. Normokalemic Periodic Paralysis.

It is an extremely rare form. Unlike the other two forms, here muscle weakness may last for 7 – 14 days and the paralysis is never complete. Muscle tone is decreased diffusely, tendon reflexes are weakened or absent. Sometimes hypertrophy of the calves develops. Biochemical tests detect normal level of serum sodium, potassium and glucose. Nevertheless, infusion of sodium-containing fluids or increased intake of salt with food leads to improvement of the condition and terminates the attacks.

Diagnosis and differential diagnosis. The diagnosis is based on the clinical evolution, biochemical and electrophysiological tests. Differential diagnosis is made with acute anterior poliomyelitis, myasthenia gravis, some forms of epilepsy, muscular dystrophies, etc.

Treatment. Hypokalemic episodes benefit from parenteral or oral administration of potassium chloride solutions and Panangin. Aldosterone antagonists (Aldactone 100 – 200 mg/day) and salt and carbohydrate restriction diet are prescribed for preventing the attacks. Hyperkalemic episodes are managed by intravenous infusion of glucose-containing solutions and calcium chloride. A low-potassium diet should be followed. Normokalemic paralysis benefits from supplementing sodium chloride to food.

2.2. Myopathies in Glycogen Metabolism Disorders.

This type of myopathies results from primary defect in glycogen metabolism disturbing its degradation (glycogenoses).

There are nine glycogenoses and in five of them /II, III, IV, V and VII/ damage to skeletal muscles is observed.

2.2.1. Type II Glycogen Storage Disease (Pompe Disease).

This is an extremely severe form of glycogen storage disease, leading to death in early childhood. The pathogenesis is associated with deficiency of the enzyme acid maltase (alpha-1,4-glucosidase), which hydrolizes maltose, linear oligosaccharides and outer chains of glycogen to glucose.

Pathomorphologically degenerative changes in the liver, kidneys, heart and skeletal muscles are found. Muscle biopsy reveals significant glycogen storage. Marked myopathic changes with vacuole formations are seen under the microscope. Biochemical tests detect complete absence of acid maltase activity.

Clinical manifestations. The first signs of the disease appear at the age of about 2- 3 months. Infants experience feeding difficulties: they become easily tired and short of breath when sucking. Intense weakness of skeletal muscles becomes apparent very soon and signs of heart failure with concomitant rhythm disturbances develop. The neurologic examination demonstrates severe muscle hypotonia and in some cases muscle hypertrophy. Reflexes are usually preserved. Cerebral symptoms are not rare: impaired level of consciousness, seizures and intellectual decline.

Evolution. Children frequently suffer from intercurrent infections and usually die in a year or two.

2.2.2. Type III Glycogen Storage Disease (Forbes Disease).

This condition develops as a result of deficiency of the enzyme amylo-1,6-glucosidase in the liver and skeletal muscles, because of which debranching of glycogen reaches only the stage of limit dextrins, which accumulate in tissues. Biochemical tests reveal abnormal structure of glycogen.

The clinical manifestations are similar to those in Pompe disease, but are much milder. Moderate muscle weakness and hypotonia are evident. Frequently the liver damage is more severe and is manifested by hypoglycemia and ketosis.

The diagnosis is confirmed by biochemical testing which proves deficiency of amylo-1,6-glucosidase in skeletal muscle and liver biopsy specimen.

2.2.3. Type V Glycogen Storage Disease (Mc Ardle Disease).

Synonyms. Aphosphorilasis muscularis, glycogenosis muscularis.

Autosomal recessive pattern of inheritance is supposed. X-linked transmission is also possible because predominantly males are affected.

Pathomorphologic examination reveals increased amount of glycogen in skeletal muscles and decreased activity of muscle phosphorylase which is responsible for glycogen degradation.

Clinical manifestations. The disease develops in childhood. The initial symptoms are easy muscle tiredness, weakness and muscle pain after physical exercises. Myoglobinuria may be detected during such crises. In some cases hypotrophy of proximal muscles might develop. The clinical course is of varying severity. Some patients are able to alleviate their muscle complaints by overcoming the so-called "dead point" during exercise ("second-wind" phenomenon).

The diagnosis is supported by muscle biopsy, EMG and histochemical tests which confirm the absence of myophosphorylase.

Treatment. Glucose and fructose intake prior to physical exercises offer a good alternative.

2.2.4. Type IV Glycogen Storage Disease (Andersen Disease) and Type VII   Glycogen Storage Disease.

They are extremely rare. Here the cardinal symptom is liver impairment, especially in Andersen disease, and muscle damage is less pronounced.

2.3. Myopathies in Lipid Metabolism Disturbances.

Some lipid metabolism disturbances may lead to increased lipid storage in muscles and development of myopathies.

2.3.1. Myopathy in Carnitine Deficiency.

Carnitine is a substance that takes part in fatty acid transportation from the cytoplasm into the mitochondria where beta-oxidation is accomplished. The enzyme carnitine palmityl transferase participates in this process.

The pathogenesis of carnitine myopathy is related to deficiency of carnitine or the enzyme which destroys it. This leads to defective utilization of fatty acids, which are esterified with glycerol in the sarcoplasm, and triglycerides or neutral fatty acids accumulate in myofibrils.

Pathomorphology. Significant storage of fatty vacuoles and degeneration is seen in muscle fibers type I.

Clinical manifestations. The course of carnitine myopathy varies in severity: it is mild in some patients, whereas in others it may lead to significant disability and lethal outcome. In most cases the onset is in the first decade of life. Muscle hypotonia and cramps, provoked by physical strain, are observed. Proximal muscles of the limbs, neck, face and trunk are affected predominantly. Liver functions are impaired too.

The diagnosis is based on muscle biopsy and biochemical tests that confirm carnitine deficiency.

Treatment. Increased consumption of carbohydrates prior to physical exercises offers a beneficial effect on symptoms.

2.3.2. Malignant Hyperthermia.

The disease is inherited in autosomal dominant pattern.

The pathobiochemical basis of the disease is increased sensitivity of the sarcoplasmic reticulum to some inhalational anesthetics (halothan) and myorelaxants (succinylcholine), as a result of which calcium metabolism in myofibrils is impaired and muscle rigidity occurs. Activation of calcium-myosine ATPase leads to significant intensification of oxidative and glycolytic phosphorylation, resulting in hyperthermia and acidosis.

Clinical manifestations. The condition might be subclinical for a long period of time with mild hypothrophy of lower limb muscles, gait changes and weakening of tendon reflexes. Exposure to general anesthetics leads to severe and dramatic symptoms of hyperthermia (41 – 42°C), cramps, severe muscle rigidity, tachypnea, cyanosis and metabolic acidosis. Muscle necrosis and myoglobinuria and eventually acute renal failure might be detected. CPK is significantly increased.

Treatment. Patients at risk should be premedicated with Dantrolene 4- 8 mg/kg in 3 doses prior to anesthesia. During an attack besides Dantrolene, barbiturates, osmotic diuretics, glucose, antiarrhythmic agents and hypothermia are also applied.

3. Myotonic Disturbances (Myotonic Myopathies).

Myotonias are a heterogenous group of inherited muscular disorders characterized by muscle tone disturbances, manifested in difficult muscle relaxation following voluntary contraction.

It is considered that the pathogenesis of myotonia /70/ is based on disturbances affecting the sarcoplasmic membrane or the muscular part of the motor unit.

There are inherited myotonias (slowly progressing forms), myotonic syndromes (in some myopathies and CNS disorders) and pseudomyotonias (in internal diseases).

3.1. Congenital Myotonia.

Synonyms. Myotinia congenita (Thomsen disease), hereditary myotonia, hereditary ataxia.

Frequency. 0.3 – 0.7:100 000 of the population.

Etiology and pathogenesis. Congenital myotonia is inherited in autosomal dominant pattern. A characteristic pathophysiological finding is repetitive depolarization of the sarcolema. Provoking factors include cold, hunger, hormonal disbalance, etc. /33/.

Pathomorphology. Biopsy specimen reveals hypertrophy of separate muscle fibers and reduced size of fibers type II. Electronic microscopy finds moderate hypertrophy of sarcoplasmic reticulum, changes in the shape and size of mitochondria and widening of the telephragm and myofibrils.

Clinical manifestations. Myotonic spasms are the cardinal symptom: abnormal muscle relaxation following voluntary contraction. The initial signs are present at birth. Poor sucking, myotonic reaction of the orbicular ocular muscles and positive Graefe's sign are observed. A hand flexed in fist remains this way for a long time despite the patient's will to open it. Repetitive voluntary contractions make myotonic events gradually fade away. Another cardinal clinical manifestation is increased mechanical excitation of muscles. Percussion with the reflex hammer over the muscle or pinching it causes muscle contraction. Percussion over the tongue results in a deep furrow: "tongue symptom". Because of diffuse muscle hypertrophy, patients look athletic. Muscles are consistent, stiff on palpation, but muscle strength is decreased. Tendon reflexes are normal, but in case of severe myotonia they are decreased.

Diagnosis and differential diagnosis. The diagnosis is based on the data from the genealogic analysis, the clinical manifestations (myotonic syndrome and athletic appearance) and EMG which gives evidence of a myotonic reaction. Differential diagnosis is made with the other forms of myotonia, pseudohypertrophic forms of PMD, tetanoid conditions, paroxysmal myoplegia, etc.

Evolution. The course is slowly progressive. Work capacity is preserved for a long period of time.

Treatment. Diphenin is used at a dose of 0.1 – 0.2 g 3 times a day, Hydantoin, Diazepam and Novocainamide. The aim is to suppress monosynaptic and polysynaptic conduction it the central nervous system.

3.2. Dystrophic Myotonia.

Synonyms. Steinert disease, Curschmann-Batten-Steinert disease, dystrophia myotonica, myotonia atrophica.

Frequency. 2.5 -5:100 000 of the population.

Etiology and pathogenesis. Transmitted in autosomal dominant pattern. The pathologic gene is localized in chromosome 19. The metabolism of the enzyme myotonin-protein kinase is disturbed. Adult males and females are equally affected.

Pathomorphology. Areas of hyperthrophy and atrophy are seen in muscle fibers and expansion of connective and adipose tissue in place of the myofibrils. Electron microscopy reveals pathologic changes in mitochondria and destruction of the myofibrillar apparatus and sarcoplasmic reticulum.

Clinical manifestations. The onset is usually at the age of 10 – 20 years. Coexistence of myotonic, dystrophic, neuroendocrine, cardiovascular and often mental disturbances is typical. Myotonic symptom complex is manifested by tonic spasms localized in the fingers, tongue, chewing muscles and extensors. Abnormal muscle contraction is evident when percussing over the thenar and the edge of the tongue. Dystrophic syndrome is characterized by pathologic muscle tiredness, weakness and muscle atrophies localized predominantly in facial, cervical and distal limb muscles. Because of the atrophies the patients' appearance is typical: there is poor head control, the face is amimic – "myopathic face", the hand looks like a monkey hand and the gait becomes "steppage" (foot drop gait). Muscle tone is decreased and tendon reflexes disappear early. Neuroendocrine disturbances in males include cryptorchidism and impotence, and affected females have ovarial dysfunction. Cardiovascular disturbances are always present. These include arrhythmia, AV block, etc. Mental symptoms are manifested as progressive dementia, mental retardation, sometimes acute psychotic attacks.

Diagnosis and differential diagnosis. The diagnosis is based on the genealogic analysis, the characteristic symptom complex and several instrumental tests. EMG reveals myotonic bursts of increasing frequency when a single stimulus is applied. ECG shows evidence of cardiomyopathy with rhythm disturbances, and CT demonstrates progressive brain atrophy. The final diagnosis is based on the evidence received from muscle biopsy. The disease must be distinguished from congenital myotonia, neural muscular atrophy, myotonic forms of PMD, etc.

Evolution. Slow progression.

Treatment. No pathogenic therapy is available. Anabolic steroids, sex hormones and vitamin E are applied. Corticosteroids are useful in some patients. Myotonic manifestations are improved by administration of membrane stabilizing substances: Phenytoin, Ajmaline, etc.

3.3. Paramyotonia and Other Rare Forms.

3.3.1. Congenital Paramyotonia.

Synonyms. Eulenburg's disease, hereditary cold paralysis, intermittent congenital myotonia.

Inherited in dominant pattern.

Clinical manifestations. Myotonic symptoms present when patients are exposed to cold and disappear with warming. As the pathologic process progresses, secondary muscular atrophies develop, but they are not obligatory.

Diagnosis and differential diagnosis. Diagnosing this form is similar to diagnosing the other forms of myotonia. As a differential diagnosis one should consider neuromyotonia (Isaac`s syndrome). In this condition there is stiffness of all facial and skeletal muscles, which does not disappear while sleeping and getting warmed, but only with application of myorelaxants. There is concurrent hyperhidrosis, increased basal metabolic rate and areflexia. EMG shows no myotonic reaction. Stiffman syndrome also includes stiffness of axial, cervical and proximal limb muscles. Facial muscles, however, are not affected. EMG shows no myotonic features /50/.

Evolution. The course is long and more favorable compared to congenital and dystrophic myotonia.

Treatment. It is not different from that in other myotonias.

Chapter IX

GENETIC COUNSELING, PROGNOSIS AND WORK
CAPACITY OF PATIENTS SUFFERING FROM HEREDITARY
DEGENERATIVE DISEASES OF THE NERVOUS SYSTEM

I. Genetic Counseling.

In cases of genetic diseases of the nervous system usually parents who seem to be healthy seek advice from a specialist for the condition of a sick child or other family member. Therefore extending prospective counsels is needed: counseling young people before getting married or counseling husband and wife before giving birth of their first child.

The clinico-genealogic method is the main method in medico-genetic counseling. It makes possible diagnosing the disease, establishing the pattern of transmission in the family, distinguishing the genome pathology from the phenocopy. The genealogic tree is studied. The proband and his/her close relatives are examined using suitable clinical and additional diagnostic methods. The genetic card includes detailed information about the patient, his/her parents, children and siblings. It is desirable to gather data about the relatives from at least 3 or 4 generations.

After establishing the pattern of inheritance (dominant or recessive) it is important to calculate the coefficient of penetrance of the pathologic gene (the latter very rarely reaches 100%). For example, in cases of complete expression of the dominant gene the risk for the proband`s children to have the disease is 50%; if the coefficient of penetrance is around 50% the risk is 25%, etc. Estimation of the risk in autosomal recessive diseases when the parents' genotypes are already known, is based on Mendelian laws (1:1:2).

Marriages between patients suffering from recessive diseases involving the nervous system are in fact rare due to the occurring severe abnormalities. If, however, the second spouse is genetically healthy, the children from such a marriage will be phenotypically healthy despite caring the pathologic gene. In the future they should not marry their relatives even if they appear healthy.

One of the reasons for spreading of hereditary diseases is the isolated location of some towns and villages and the resulting consanguinity or marriages based on financial or politic interests. In such cases children suffering from autosomal recessive diseases are often born (Friedreich's ataxia, torsion dystonia, etc.), because the related parents might be heterozygote carriers of the same pathologic gene, inherited from common predecessors. This is probably the way of determination of the level of consanguinity between spouses. In marriages between siblings it is ¼, in marriage between uncles and nephews it is 1/8, etc.

Therefore diagnosing practically asymptomatic heterozygote carriers of the pathologic gene is important for genetic counseling, and this requires clinical, biochemical and electrophysiological tests. Thus in healthy appearing relatives of the proband suffering from hereditary ataxia mild muscle hypotonia, latent nystagmus, positive Romberg sign, etc. are noted. Some biochemical changes - insignificantly decreased adrenaline and noradrenalin excretion - are found in phenotypically healthy relatives of patients with Parkinson Disease. The increased activity of serum creatine phosphokinase (over 5 UI) is a sign of caring the pathologic gene in X-linked myopathy (Duchenne type). Some EMG changes in healthy appearing relatives of patients with Strümpell disease can be interpreted as an initial manifestation of the condition.

Many other factors, besides the risk of giving birth to a sick child, must be considered: the characteristics of the disease evolution in the family, the life expectancy, etc. The negative influence of some exogenous factors must also be kept in mind: infections, birth trauma, etc. They can exert an unfavorable effect upon the penetrance and expression of the pathologic gene and the clinical course as a whole.

After considering the influence of all these and many other factors, genetic counseling must be able to provide an answer to the question whether a marriage between the risk groups is appropriate and whether interruption of pregnancy is required. The answer to these questions is complex and depends both on the correct drawing of the genealogic tree and on the performance of some modern biochemical methods such as examination of amniotic fluid in pregnant women, in whose family there are patients with hereditary degenerative diseases of the nervous system.

2. Prognosis of Degenerative Diseases of the Nervous System.

It is generally unfavorable with a few exceptions. Despite the progress achieved in treating diseases of the nervous system such as Parkinson disease, hepatolenticular degeneration, some forms of progressive muscular dystrophies, etc., therapy in most cases is far from effective. As a rule, the recessive forms of this group of diseases follow a more severe course than the dominant conditions.

3. Work Capacity.

Work capacity is temporarily or permanently lost in the most patients.

In relatively milder forms of scapulohumeral and distal myopathy, Parkinson Disease, neural muscular atrophy and Strümpell disease, patients with late onset of the disorder are capable to work for a long period of time if their job is not associated with intensive physical exertion. These patients should not overwork themselves physically and must avoid contact with toxins. Patients suffering from Thomsen myotonia should not practice jobs associated with rapid and continuing movements: turners, fitters, etc. In other cases (myoclonus epilepsy, hereditary ataxia, juvenile form of myopathy) work capacity is lost from the initial stages of the disorder. Patients suffering from Strüpmell disease and myopathies, however, can preserve the capability of performing precise movements and intellectual occupations related to reading, writing, calculations, etc. for a long period of time. In such cases IIIrd invalidity group can be assigned and with disease progression it can be changed to IInd and Ist group. In cases of autosomal recessive and more severe forms of hereditary degenerative diseases of the nervous system Ist invalidity group can be established from the beginning.

ABBREVIATIONS USED

ATP – Adenosine triphosphate
GABA – Gamma-amino butyric acid
DNA – Deoxyribonucleic acid
EEG – Electroencephalogram
EMG – Electromyogram
CT – Computer tomography
CPK – Creatine phosphokinase
PMN – Peripheral motor neuron
HSMN – Hereditary motor-sensory neuropathy
CMN – Central motor neuron
CN – Cranial nerves
MRI – Magnetic resonance imaging

CONTENTS

Orthochromatic Leukodystrophy.

Rare forms / Globoid Cell Leukodystrophy, Peliceaus-Merzbacher Disease/.

Leukodystrophies with Secondary Disturbance of Myelin Metabolism and Structure. Aminoacidurias. Phenylketonuria.

Other Metabolic Disturbances Affecting the Nervous System.

Syndromes in Disturbed Cholesterol Metabolism.

Hand-Schüller-Cristian Disease.

Van Bogaert Cerebrotendinous Xanthomatosis.

Syndromes of Disturbed Pyrine Metabolism.

Lesch-Nyhan Syndrome.

Chapter V. SYSTEMIC ATROPHIES OF CORTICOSPINAL AND CORTICOBULBAR MOTOR NEURON SYSTEMS. - I. Manchev

Amyotrophic Lateral Sclerosis.

Progressive Bulbar Paralysis. Fazio-Londe Syndrome.

Strümpell Disease.

Chapter VI. HEREDITARY DEGENERATIVE DISEASES OF SPINAL MOTONEURONS - Spinal Muscular Atrophies. - I. Manchev

Infantile Form /Werdnig-Hoffmann/.

Infantile Chronic Form /Intermediate/.

Juvenile Form /Kugelberg-Welander/.

Distal Type.

Spinal Muscular Atrophy in Adults.

Chapter VII. HEREDITARY POLYNEUROPATHIES /Charcot-Marie-Tooth Disease/. - I. Manchev

Hereditary Motor and Sensory Polyneuropathies Type I, II, III.

Hereditary Sensory and Autonomic Neuropathies.

Hereditary Polyneuropathies with Metabolic Disturbance.

Chapter VIII. HEREDITARY MYOPATHIES. - I. Manchev

Progressive Muscular Dystrophies.

X-recessive Forms.

Girdle Forms /"Limb-Girdle" Forms/.

Facioscapulohumeral Form.

Scapuloperoneal Forms.
Congenital, Structural and Other Rare Forms.
Metabolic Myopathies.
Myotonic Disturbances /Myotonic Myopathies/.
Congenital Myotonia.
Dystrophic Myotonia.
Paramyotonia and Other Rare Forms.

Chapter IX. GENETIC COUNSELING, PROGNOSIS AND WORK
CAPACITY OF PATIENTS SUFFERING FROM HEREDITARY
DEGENERATIVE DISEASES OF THE NERVOUS SYSTEM
- I. Manchev

REFERENCES:

1. Badalian L.O., Jurba L.T., Vsevoljcsaia H.M. Handbook of Pediatric Neurology. Kiev, "Zdarovia", 1980.
2. Bojinov S. Polyneuritis and polyneuropathies. M., Med. And Health., 1984.
3. Georgiev Iv., Nachev., Bojinov S. Lipidosis and Leucodystrophies. In book : Synthetic Neurology. Edited by S.Bojinov, Iv. Georgiev, M.,Med. And Health., 1981, 113-130.
4. Georgiev Iv., Karamalakov L. Cortical and extrapyramidal syndromes and dystrophies. In book: Handbook of Neurology. Edited by D. Hadjiev, Iv. Georgiev, M. Med. And Health, 1988, 193-220.
5. Gusev E.I., Grechko B.E., Burd G.S. Hereditary neurology disease. In book : Neurology disease. Moskow, "Medicine", 1988, 583-623.
6. Iordanov B., Yankov Y. Rear syndromes and disease nervous system. M. Med. And Health, 1979.
7. Kerekovski Iv. Pediatric neurology. M., Med. And Health, 1982.
8. Martinov J.S. Heredodegenerative diseases. In book: Neurology disease. Moskow, "Medicine", 1988.
9. Cucer M.B. Pediatric clinical neuropathology. Moskow. "Medicine", 1978.
10. Shmidt E.V., Vereshchagin N.V., Bragina L.K. at al. Synopsis of neurology. Edited by E.V. Shmidt, Moskow, "Medicine", 1989.
11. Aminoff M.J. Electromyography in Clinical Practice. 2nd ed. Churchill Livingstone, 1987.
12. Asbury A.K., Gilliatt R.W. (ed) Peripheral Nerve Disorders. Butterwort&Co Publ., London, 1984.
13. Bird T.D., Cedelbaum S., Valpey R.W.et al. Familial degeneration of the basal ganglia with acanthocytosis: a

clinical, neuropathological and neurochemical study. Ann. of Neurology, 1978, 3, 253-258.

14. Bird T.D., Ott G., Giblett E.R. Evidence for lincage of Charcot-Marie-Tooth neuropathy to the Duffy locus on chromosome 1. Am.J. of Human Genetics, 1982, 34, 388-394.

15. Bonifati V., et al. Clinical and genetic features of familial Parkinson's disease. New trends in clin. Neuropharmacology, 1994, 8,69.

16. Bosch E.P., Hart M.N. Late adult – onset metachromatic leucodystrophy. Archives of Neurology, /Chicago/, 1978, 35, 475-477.

17. Boysen G., Galasi G., Kamienska Z. et al. Familial amyloidosis with cranial neuropathy and corneal lattice Dystrophy. J. of Neurol., Neurosurg. And Psych.., 1979, 42, 1020 – 1030.

18. Brady R.O., Uhlendorf B.W., Jacobson C. B. Fabry's disease: antenatal detection. Science, 1971, 172, 174-175.

19. Buchthal F., Behse F. Peroneal muscular atrophy and related diseorders. In: Clinical manifestacion as related to biopsy findings, nerve conduction and electromyography. Brain, 1977, 100, 41-66.

20. Calne D., Langston G. Etiology of Parkinson's disease. Lancet, 1983, 2, 1457-1459.

21. Chokroverty S., Duvoisin R., Sachdeo R. et al. Neurophysiologic study of olivopontocerebellar atrothy with or without glutamate dehydrogenase deficiency. Neurology, 1985, 35, 652-659.

22. Contrady S. et al. Abnormal distribution of lead in amyotrophic lateral sclerosis. Reestimation of lead in the cerebrospinal fluid. G. Neurol. Sci., 1980, 48, 413-418.

23. Chauldry V. et al. Multifocal motor neuropathy: response to human immune globulin. Ann. Neurol., 1993, 33, 237-242.

24. Delank H.W. Neurologie. Ferdinand Ence Verlag, Stuttgart, 1994.

25. Dubisky R.M. Tremor and dystonya. In: Handbook of Tremor Desorders. Eds. Findley L.G., Koller W.C., Marcel Dekker Inc., New York, 1995, 405-410.
26. Dyck P.G. Peripheral neuropathy. 3rd et., Saunders, 1993.
27. Elder G.H. et al. The primary enzyme defect in hereditary corpoporphyria. Lancet, 1976, 2, 1217-1219.
28. Engel W.K. Introduction to the myopathies. In: Sciantific approaches to Clin. Neurol. Ed.E. S. Goldenson and S.A.Appel. Philadelphia, 1977, 1555, 1571.
29. Farpour H., Mahloudji M. Familial cerebrotendinous xanthomatosis. Report of a new family and review of the literature. Arch. Neurol., 1975, 32, 223-225.
30. Feero W.G. et al. Hypercalemic periodic paralysis: Rapid molecular diagnosis and relationship of genotype to phenotype in 12 families. Neurology, 1993, 43, 668-673=
31. Fishbeck K.H., Garbern J.V. Fascioscapulohumeral muscular dystrophy defect identified. Nature Genet, 1992, 2, 3-4.
32. Fishbeck K.H. The mechanism of myotonic dystrophy. Ann. Neurol., 1994, 35, 255-256.
33. Gibb W. et al. Cortical Levy body dementia: clinical feature and classification. J. Neurol. Neurosurg. And Psych., 1988, 51, 752-754. Goodman R.M. Genetic Disorders of Man. Boston, LittleBrown, 1970, 1009-1023.
34. Guiloff R.J. et al. Evidence of lincage of type 1 hereditary motor and sensory neuropathy with the Duffi Locus on chromosome 1. Ann. of Human Genetics. 1982, 46, 25-27.
35. Gutmann D.H., Fishbeck K.H. Molecular biology of Dushenne and Becker`s muscular dystrophy: Clinical applications. Ann. Neurol., 1989, 26, 189-194.
36. Harberg B., Lyon G. Pooled European series of hereditary peripheral neuropathies in infancy and childhood. /EFCNS/, Neuropediatrics, 1981, 12, 9-17.
37. Hahn A. et al. A variant form of metachromatic leucodystrophy without arylsulphatase deficiency. Ann. of Neurology, 1982, 12, 33-36.
38. Harding A.E. Friedreih`s ataxia: a clinical and genetic study of 90 families with an analysis of early diagnostic criteria

and intrafamilia clustering of clinical features. Brain, 1981, 104, 589-620.

39. Harding A.E., Thomas P.K. The clinical features of hereditary motor and sensory types 1 and 2. Brain, 1980, 103, 259-280.

40. Harding A.E., Mathews S., Jones S. et al. Spinocerebellar degeneration associated with a selective defect of vitamin E absorbtion. N. Engl. J. Med., 1985, 313, 32-35.

41. Herbert P.N., Gotto A.M., Friedrickson D.S. Familial lipoprotein deficiency/ abetalipoproteinemia, hypobetalipoproteinemia, and Tangier disease/, In: The metabolic basis of Inherited disease, et. J.B.Stanbury, J.B.Wyngaarden, D.S.Friedrickson, New York, McGrow Hill, 1978, 545-588.

42. Holmes G.L., Shauwitz B.A. Strumpell`s pure familial spastic paraplegia: Case study and revew of the literature. J. Neurol., Neurosurg., Psychiatry, 1977, 40, 1003-1008.

43. Killian J.M., Kloepfer H.W. Homosygous expretion of a dominant mutant gene for Charcot-Marie-Tooth neuropathy. Ann. Neurology, 1979, 5, 515-522.

44. Kohler W.C., Hubble J.P., Busenbark K.L. Esencial tremor. In: Other neurodegenerative Disease. Ed. Calne D.B., Saunders W.B., Philadelphia, 1994, 717-742.

45. Kugelberg E. Chronic proximal /pseudomyopathic/ spinal muscular atrophy. In: Hanndbook of Clinical Neurology, v.22, ed. Vinken P.J., Bruyn, Amsterdam, 1975, 67-80.

46. Lewis R.A., Grunnel M.L., Zimmerman A.W. Peripheral nerve demyelination in Cockayne`s syndrome. Muscle and Nerve, 1982, 5, 557-561.

47. Lewis R.A., Sumner A.J. The electrodiagnostic distinctions between chronic familial and acquired demyelinating neuropathies. Neurology. 1982, 592-596.

48. Lorish T.H., Thorstenson G., Howard F.M. In: Stiff-man syndrome updated. Mayo Clin. Rroc., 1989, 64, 629-636.

49. Less A.J. Tics and related disorders. Churchill Livingstone, London, 1985.

50. Mc Leod J.G., Ewans W.A. Peripheral neuropathy in spinocerebellar degenerations. Muscle and Nerve, 1981, 1, 51-61.
51. Mendel J.R. et al. Randomized, double –blid six-month trial of prednisone in Duchenne`s muscular dystrophy. N. Engl. J. Med., 1989, 320, 1592-1597.
52. Mulder D.W. The Diagnosis and Treatment of Amyotrophic Lateral Sclerosis. Boston. Houghton Mifflin Professional Publishers, 1979.
53. Muller D.P., Loyd J.K., Bird A.C. Longoterm management of abetalipoproteinemia. Possible role of vitamin A. Archives of Disease in Childhood, 1977, 52, 209-214.
54. Mitsumoto H., Sliman R.G. Schafer et al. Moptor neuron disease and adult hexosaminidase. A deficiency in two families evidence for multisystem degeneration. Ann. Neurol., 1985, 17, 378-385.
55. Murray T.J. Congenital sensory neuropathy. Brain, 1973, 96, 378, 394.
56. Mustajoki P. Variegate porphyria. Ann. of Int. Med. 1978, 89, 328-244.
57. Nordborg C., Conradi N., Sounranrer P.A. A new type of non-progressive sensory neuropathy in chidren with atypical dysautonomia. Acta Neuropatholobica. Berlin, 1981, 55, 135-141.
58. Nukuda H., Poolock M., Haas L.F. The clinical spectrum of type II hereditary sensory neuropathy. Brain, 1982, 105, 647-665.
59. Ohnishi A., Sato Y., Nagara Het al. Neurogenetic muscularatrophy and low density of large myelinated fibres of sural nerve of chorea-acantocytosis. J. of Neurol. Neurosurg. And Psych., 1981, 44, 645-648.
60. O`Neill B.P. et al. Adrenoleukodystrophy: Clinical and Biochemical manifestacion in carries. Neurology, 1984, 34, 798-801.
61. Ouvrier R.A. et al. Hereditary motor and sensory neuropathy of neuronal type with onset in early childhood. J. of Neurol., Sci., 1981, 51, 181-197.

62. Ouvrier R.A., Mc Leod J.G., Couchin T.E. Friedreich's ataxia: Early detection ond progression of peripheral nerve abnormalities. J. Neurol. Sci., 1982, 55, 137-145.
63. Pearn J. Classification of spinal muscular artopathies. Lancet, 1980, 919-922.
64. Pearn J.H., Hugson P., Walton J.N. A clinical and genetic study of spinal muscular atrophy of adult onset. The autosomal recessive form as a discreate antity. Brain, 1978, 101, 591-606.
65. Perkin G.D. Diagnostic Tests in Neurology . Chapman and Hall, London, 1988.
66. Petty R.K., Harding A.E., Mogran-Hughes J.A. The clinical features of mitochondrial myopathy. Brain, 1986, 109, 915-938.
67. Plaitakis A., Nicklas W., Desnick R. Glutamate dehydrogenase deficiency in three patients with spinocerebellar syndrome. Ann. Neurol., 1980, 7, 297-303.
68. Ptacek L.J., Johnson K.J., Griggs R.C. Genetics and physiology of the myotonic muscle disorders. N. Engl. J. Med., 1993, 328, 482-489.
69. Refsum S., Stokke O., Eldjarn M. Heredopathia atactica polyneuritiformis /Refsum's disease/. In: Peripheral neuropathy. ed. P.J. Dyck, P.K. Thomas, E.H. Lambert, Philadelphia, W.B. Saunders, 1975, 868-890.
70. Ringel S.P. et al. The natural history of amyotrophic lateral sclerosis. Neurology, 1993, 43, 1316-1322.
71. Rajput A.H. Pathological and neurochemical basis of essential tremor. In: Handbook of Tremor Disorders. Ed. Findley L.J., Koller W.C.., Marcel Dekker Inc., New York, 1995, 233-244.
72. Rondot P., Bathien N. Cerebellar tremors: physiological basis and treatment. In: Handbook of Tremor Disorders. Eds. Findley L.J., Koller W.C., Marcel Dekker Inc., New York, 1995, 371-385.
73. Rossi E./ed/ Pediatrie. Georg Thieme Verlag, Stuttgart, 1989.

74. Russo L.S. Clinical and electrophysiological studies in primary lateral sclerosis. Arch. Neurol., 1982, 39, 662-664.

75. Rowland L.P. The Human Muscular Dystrophies. New York. Experta Medica, 1977.

76. Shapiro F., Bresnan M.J. Orthopedic management of childhood neuromuscular disease. Part II: Peripheral neuropathies. Friedreich`s ataxia and arthrogryposis multiplex congenital. J. of Bone and Joint Surgery, 1982, 64 A, 949-953.

77. Seigel I.M. The management of muscular dystrophy: a clinical review. Muscle and Nerve, 1978, 1, 453-460.

78. Siddique T. at al. Lincage of a gene causing familial amyotrophic lateral sclerosis to chromosome 21 and evidence of genetic-locus heterogeneity. N. Engl. J. Med., 1991, 324, 1381-1384.

79. Schapira A. Mechanisms of cell death in Parkinson`s disease. Parkinson`s disease Update Abstr., 1994, 42, 225-226.

80. Sorbi S. et al. Abnormal platelet glutamate dehydrogenase activity and activation in dominant and nondominant olivipontocerebeller atrothy. Ann., Neurol., 1986, 19, 239-245.

81. Sweiman K.F. Lipid disease of the central nervous system. In: The practice of Pediatric Neurology, ed. K.F. Sweiman and F.S. Wright, St. Louis CV, Mosby, 1975, 397-424.

82. Sweiman K.F. Mucopolysaccharoidosis. In: The Practice of Pediatric Neurology ed. K.F. Sweiman and F.S. Wright., St. Louis, VS Mosby, 1975, 424-436.

83. Taylor A.M. et al. Ataxia teleangiectasia : a human mutacion with abnormal radiation sensitivity. Nature, 1975, 258, 427-429.

84. Tishler P.V., Knighton D.J., Schumaker H.M. Screening test for intermittent acute porphyria. Lancet, 1976, 1, 303-305.

85. Vignos P.J. Rehabilitation in myopathies. In: Handbook of Clinical Neurology. V.41, part II, eds. P.J. Vinken , G.V.Bruin, S.P.Ringel, New York, North Holland, 1979, 187-226.

86. Vitek J.L., Wichmann T., De Long M.R. Current concept of basal ganglia neurophysiology relative to tremorgenesis. In: Handbook of Tremor Disorders. Eds. Findley L.J., Koller W.C., Marcel Dekker Inc., New York, 1995, 37-49.

87. Werlin S.L. et al. Diagnostic dilemmas of Wilson`s disease; diagnosis and treatment, Pediatrics, 1978, 62, 47-51.

88. Wiederholt W.C. /ed/ Therapy for neurologic disorders. J. Wiley Med. Publ., New York, 1982.

89. Willner J.P, et al. Chronic Gm2 gangliosidosis masquerading as atypical Friedreich ataxia: Clinical, morphologic and biochemical studies of nine case. Neurology, 1981, 31, 787-798.

90. Yao J.K., Dyck P.J. Lipid abnormalities in hereditary neuropathy. Part IV, Endoneurial and liver lipids of HMSN-III/Dejerine-Sottas disease/, J. of the Neurol. Sci., 1982, 52, 179-190.

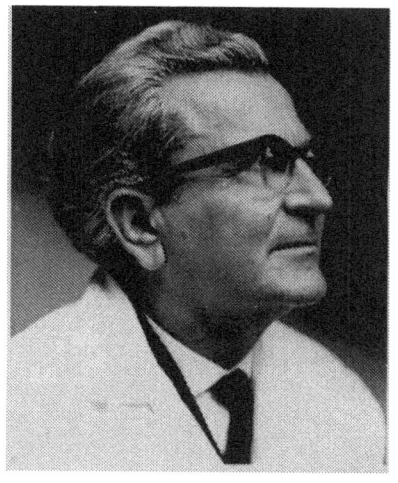

Professor D-r Ivan Georgiev graduated from the Medical faculty of Sofia University, Bulgaria. His career started in 1949 as assistant in Neurology and Psychiatry Clinic led by Professor G. Usunov and N.Shipkovenski, later as their research associate. In 1962 he become Associate Professor and in 1969 Professor in Neurology. He has been Head of Neurology department, Director of National Institute of Neurology, Psychiatry and Neurosurgery and member of the Presidium of Bulgarian Medical Academy. Main directions of his scientific career treat problems with neuroinfections, neurodystrophic processes and evolutional neurology.

He has been active member of governing bodes of: World Neurology Federation, European Association of Neurology Scientific Societies, Curatorium of Danube Symposiums of neuroscience, Bulgarian Science Union and much more.

He is associate member of Word Neurology Federation, European Association of Neurology Societies, American Psychosomatic Society, International "Pavlov`s" Society (USA), Foundation "Stroke prevention" and other's.

He is honorary member of French Neurology Society, German Neurology and Psychiatry Society and other's.